SuperPowers

Today's Affirmation...

I am :

Living to Inspire
others to Greatness

SUPER POWERS

A Busy Woman's Guide to Health & Happiness

Published by SuperPower Blue Print

Ordering Information:
Quantity sales - Special discounts are available on quantity purchases by corporations, associations, and others. For details, contact info@AditaLang.com
Orders by U.S. trade bookstores and wholesalers. Please contact info@AditaLang.com

ISBN-13: 978-1-7325351-1-4

LCCN: 2018907487

Cover design by JAS Designs
Book design and production by JAS Design and Adita Yrizarry-Lang
Chapter illustrations by JAS Design
Author photograph by JAS Design

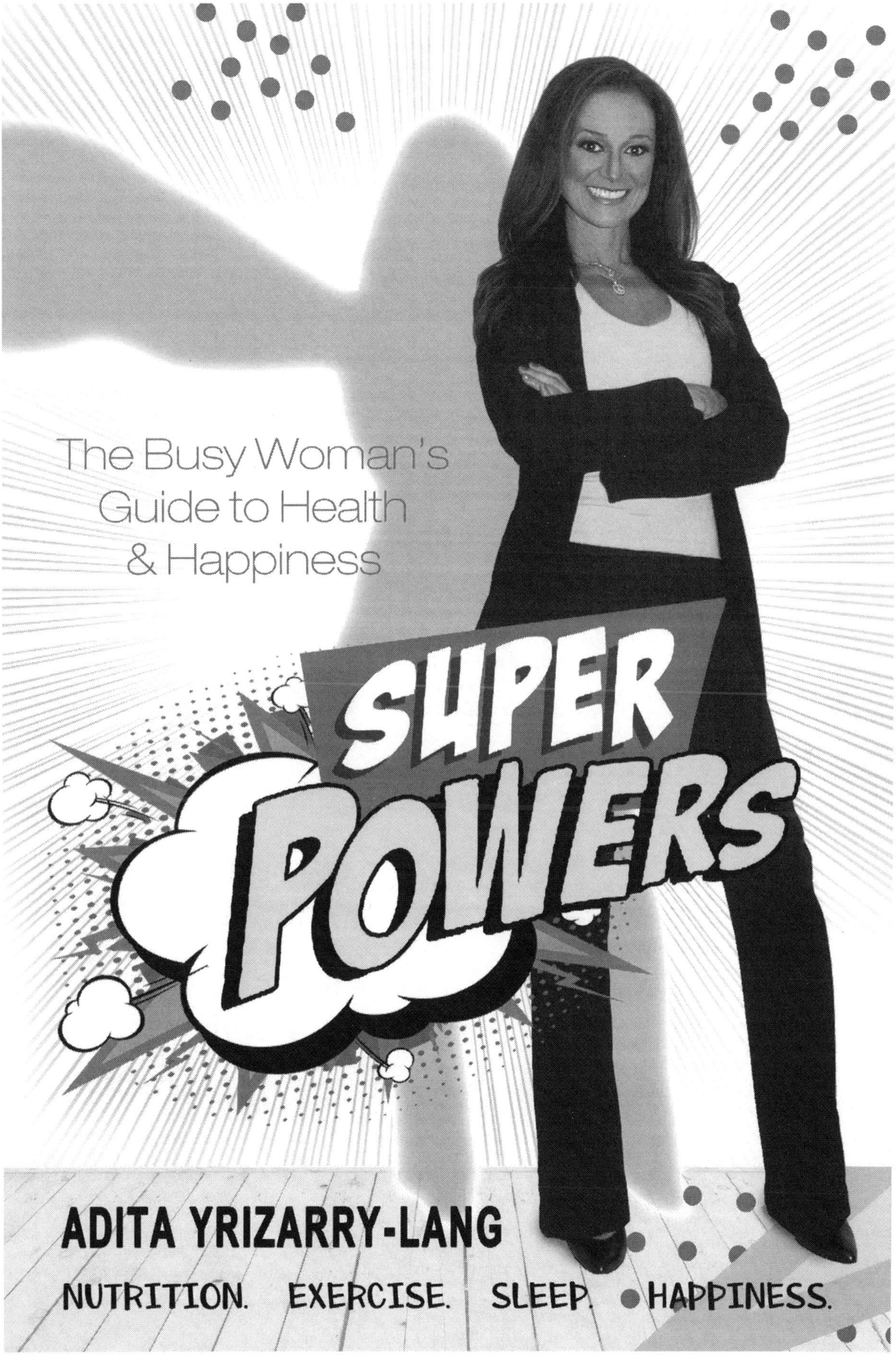
The Busy Woman's
Guide to Health
& Happiness
SUPER
POWERS
ADITA YRIZARRY-LANG
NUTRITION. EXERCISE. SLEEP. HAPPINESS.

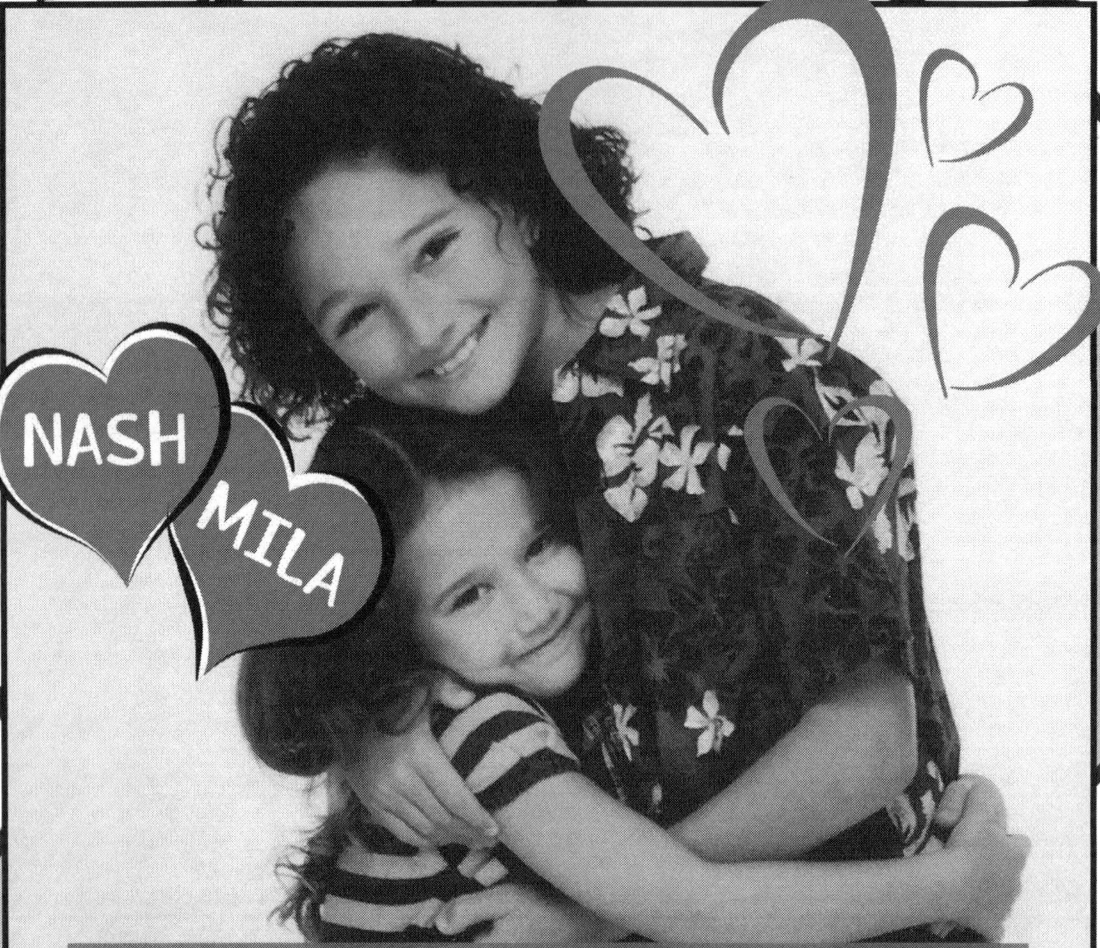

This book is dedicated to my children, Nash & Mila.

Roses are Red
Violets are Blue
You are my Blessing
And I Love YOU!

Thank you for giving me the motivation to become the very best version of myself, I will be here to inspire and love you for years to come.

KUDOS

Wow, just the idea that you are reading this book magnifies the fact that there are several people in my tribe to give thanks to. I am so blessed to have so many that inspire me and drive me to be my very best. These are my peeps and I love each and every one of you. So, as a means of keeping this to a page, yet simple enough not to bore you, here goes...

From every great person comes an amazing family that stands behind them in some way. Although my mom and I parted ways years ago, she still instilled in me a type of achievement mindset that has driven me to this day. My dad, on the other hand, has been with me throughout my life, as a cheerleader and an amazing support. He has given me the confidence to simply "try" and see where it takes me! And then, of course, there are my brothers, stepmom, aunts, uncles, cousins, and pets, all there with love and support and endless encouragement to reach for the stars.

My children have given me the strength to create a legacy, one that I can pass on to them, and one for them to shine from as well.

Then there is my tribe, those friends that inspire, encourage, and have made me who I am today. They mean the world to me and I thank them for everything they have shared with me throughout the years.

With Love and Light,

Adita

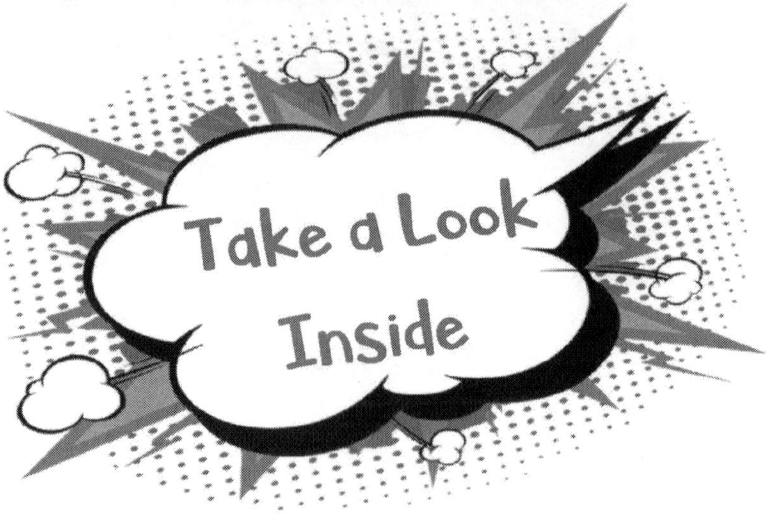
Take a Look Inside

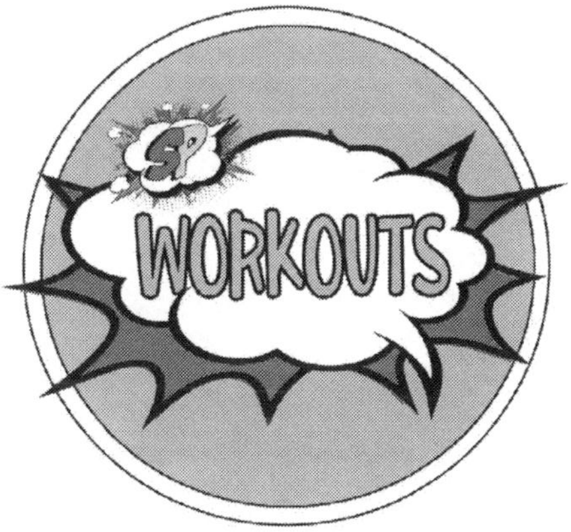
SP
WORKOUTS

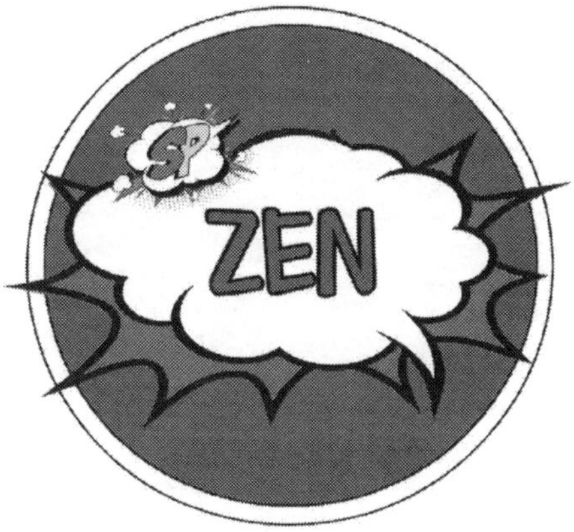
SP
ZEN

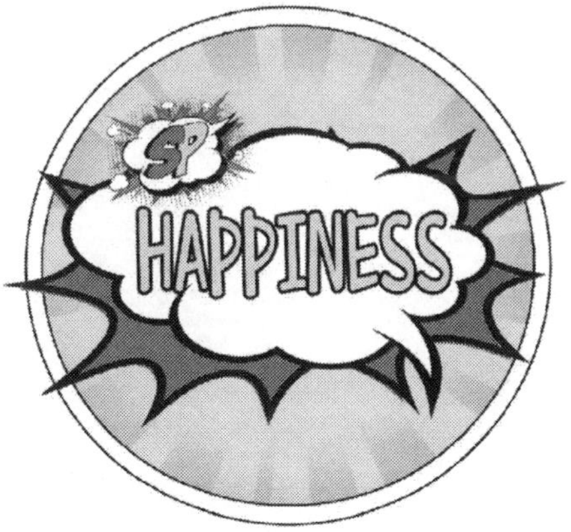
SP
HAPPINESS

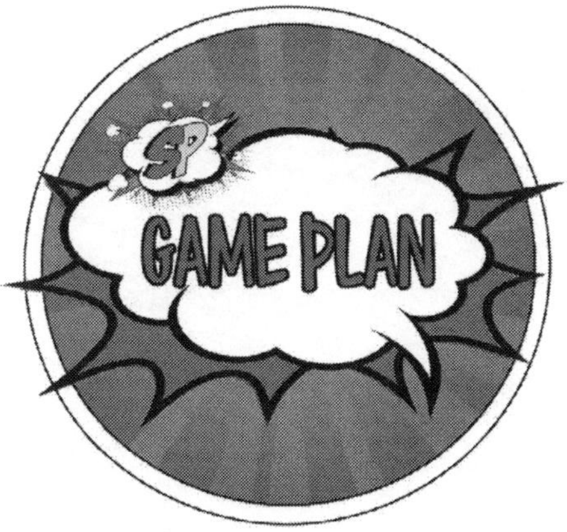
SP
GAME PLAN

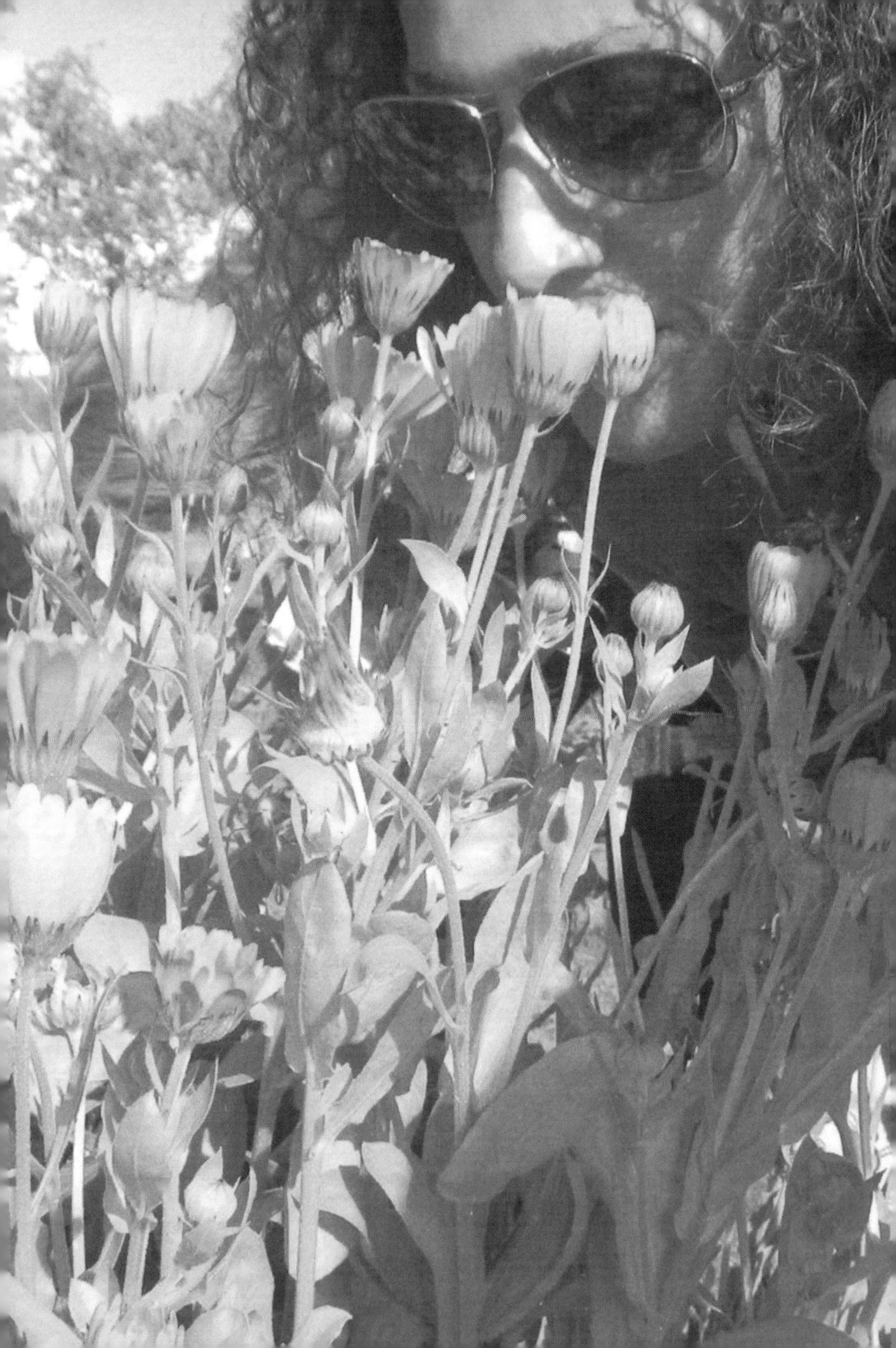

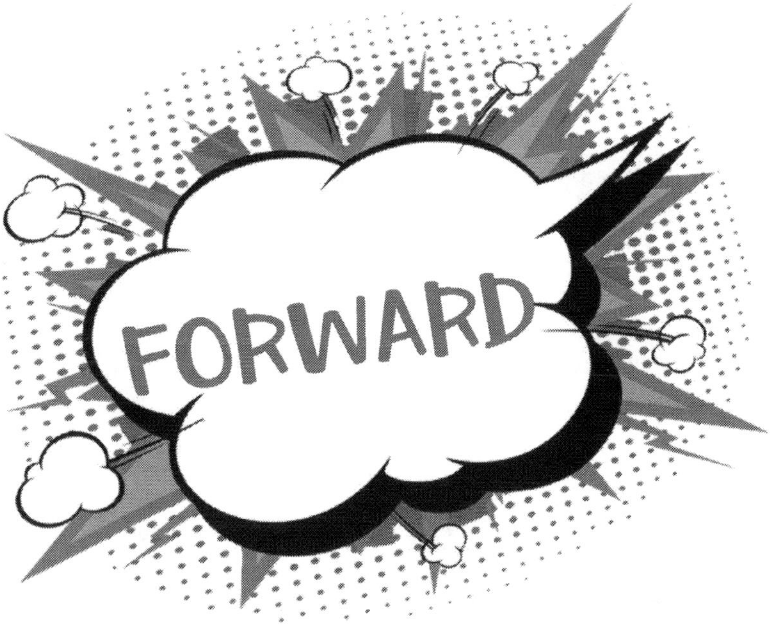

SUPERPOWERS FOREWARD - By Linda Shelton

"This book is a must for any woman who wants command of her own health and well-being, to truly live her bliss."

In the mid-80's, as aerobic workouts were trending and the fitness industry was newly developing, I met a young, bright-eyed, positive, smart and excited, newly certified fitness professional who was ready to take on the world with her recent-found education and skills. I was impressed with her tenacity, her drive to continue to learn and contribute to her community and students, her compassion, integrity and her creative, overflowing vessel of ideas. She was definitely a mover and a shaker. As an international presenter, program developer, "trainer's trainer," and part of fitness education within the fitness and wellness industry for over four decades, I'm always on the lookout for those 'with potential,' who can create sustainable, intelligent programming that has 'legs'. I watched this young woman in those days, blossom and become an amazing speaker and source of education to many.

As the industry flourished and matured, she did as well, finding new pathways to share her knowledge and change countless people's lives. She branched out into the nutrition and wellness world, studied for advanced certifications and started a new business. She became a global presenter, sharing her knowledge, venturing out of her comfort zone to challenge norms, to impart information in a fun, thought-provoking, non-intimidating way.

We hit it off, she and I, and though we live on opposite sides of the country, I'm in Los Angeles and she in Miami, we stayed in touch over the decades as fitness professionals and as friends. I became her mentor, for which I've always been grateful for her trust. As you probably have concluded by now, I have known Adita Yrizarry-Lang for about thirty years. I'm thrilled to see her latest venture and creation, Adita's first published book come to fruition.

SuperPowers: The Busy Woman's Guide to Health & Happiness perceptively written by fitness and wellness expert Adita Yrizarry-Lang, is an incredibly down to earth, DIY, self-help guide that will give you the 'super boost' you need to shift your life from blah to bliss once and for all. We, as women, think of it as a 'woman's dilemma'—constantly juggling career, home, family, kids, personal needs and wants for priority on our daily to do lists. It's a societal issue and there will never be enough time, unless we make it and take it!

This book is a brilliant and realistic example of how you can always adjust and go with the flow, create positive life changes and have it all! You'll find every chapter is filled with tips, tools and step by step action items to give every woman the confidence and knowledge to begin to take charge of her life. This well organized and thoughtful book is written in a positive, up-front and fresh tone, without the lecture. The simple, easy to follow information throughout provides a template for how you can re-gain your SuperPowers---self-confidence, self-awareness and control and begin to engage in your life in a more pro-active, mindful and courageous way. It's time to *unleash the lioness* in you!

Adita puts the reality check out there regarding how to acquire and maintain a healthy and fit lifestyle to make it work for YOU! The skillful use of color, interactive illustrations and simple phrases definitely will draw you in. Adita, in down to earth, positive language, identifies the challenges that most, if not all women face at some point in their lifetime. She lays out the hard research-based facts regarding the negative effects of a sedentary, harried lifestyle, when you let lack of time, stress and barriers block your SuperPowers. Her light yet educational approach, using her Four Pillars of Health, [1] Food & Nutrition, [2] Exercise & Movement, [3] Happiness & Joy, and [4] Sleep and Relaxation, makes lifestyle change feel achievable—exercise, eating, scheduling easily accessible, regardless of where you are, in your process, giving you the keys to your own freedom for a vibrant, self-managed, and holistically balanced life.

Adita is truly an inspiration in her natural ability to educate and empower others to find their SuperPowers and live the life they want and deserve. She has a warm, open style that allows her to relate to anyone. Her breadth of knowledge and expertise has served her in many fitness and wellness arenas. I can talk about all the things she has done over the span of her still growing career, as she is one of those extraordinary 'notables.' However, who she is as a person, what she gives and how she lives her life-in full gusto, with passion and heart, shines through in this book.

--Linda Shelton, Int'l fitness expert and fitness innovator, former Fitness Director of Shape Magazine, 2007 Inductee to the National Fitness Hall of Fame, Author, Video Producer/Director

"With every challenge in life comes a lesson, and with every lesson a gift!"

-Adita Lang

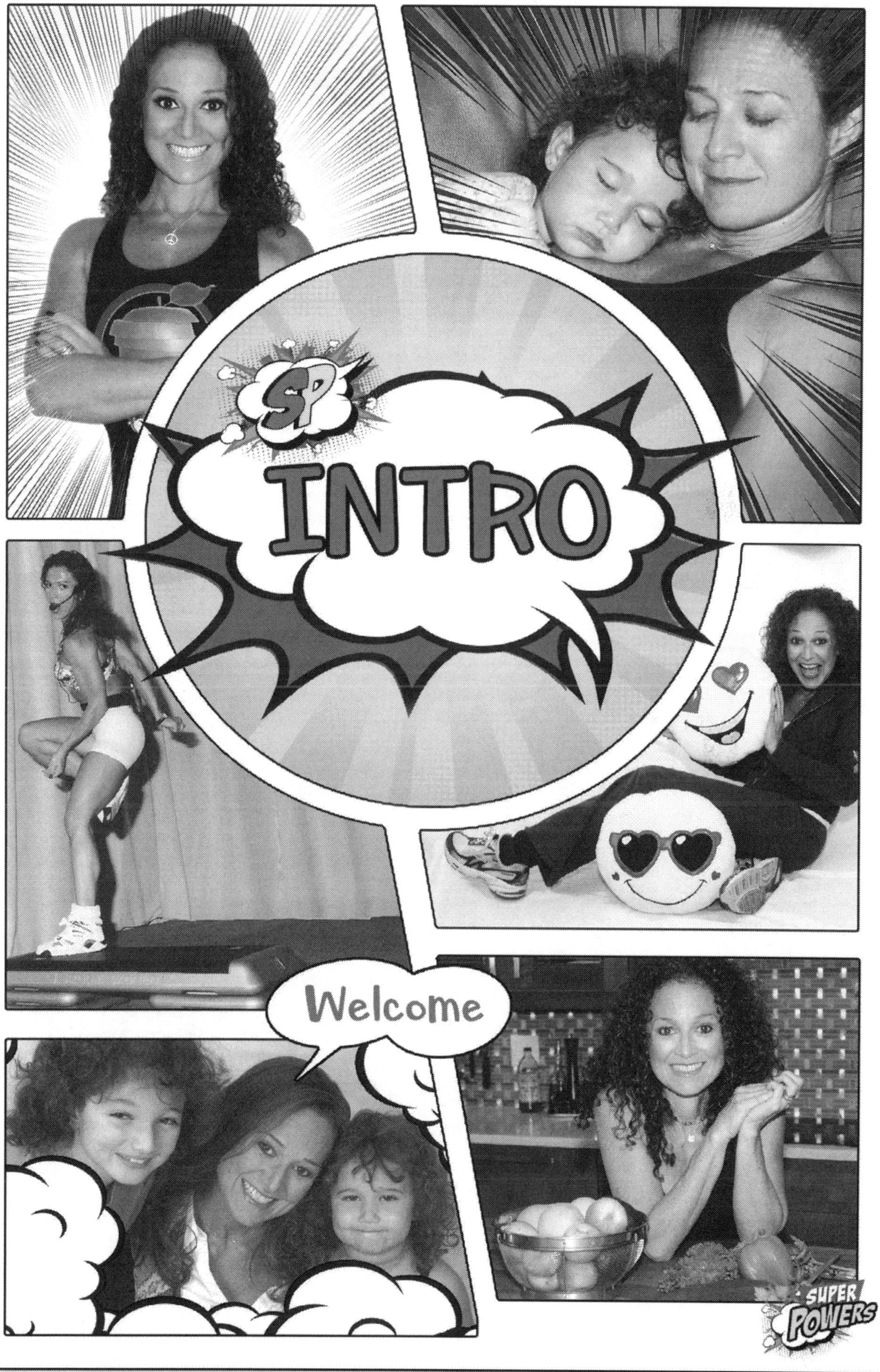
SP
INTRO
Welcome
SUPER POWERS

What Are YOUR SuperPowers Made Of?

The good old days! These were the days when I traveled, shopped, and lived life to its fullest! Many of my go-to peeps were married with kids and I had yet to settle my ass down. My SuperPowers were stronger than ever, but my health, and I'm talking "true health", was something that I really had no idea about. All I knew was that I felt great, I could lift heavy things, and I was unstoppable. We all feel this way at some point but here is the funny thing, we really have no idea what "ideal health" feels like, we only assume that if we feel good and our doctors give us that "clean bill of health", then hey, we are doing GREAT! Life is so filled with "stuff", stress "stuff", family "stuff", relationship "stuff"; you know what I'm talking about. This can and will wear us down; the key is to recognize your SuperPowers and keep them running at top performance—all the time! Funny enough, nobody ever really tells you the TRUTH about the ebb and flow of living a healthy and abundant life. It really doesn't need to be so complicated, people!

Once I settled into the norms of life—you know, the husband and kids and stuff—I literally burned the candle at both ends; one day blurred into the next and the next thing I knew my body began to challenge me in ways I never had imagined, all because I took my SuperPowers for granted again and again. Unstoppable ME was dead in her tracks and I had no idea WHY! "Dammit, I am a fitness professional, one of the healthiest people I know, how can I be lacking in energy and have a digestive system that is slower than molasses? What the..." Yup, it happens to all of us, and here is the thing; if we don't nip it in the bud it only gets worse. And honestly, if it gets worse and we don't act on it, it's only going to take longer to resolve. Your energy, health, and vivaciousness for life are those things that give you SuperPowers. We have them at every age; it simply depends on how much importance we want to give them.

Are your SuperPowers tuned up to perfection or are they lagging in response time? Did you even realize that you have them? Well, of course you do, it's just a matter of revving them back up to shine like never before! So no worries; by the time I'm done with you, you will reignite yourself without skipping a beat! Now, if you're not too sure if your current powers are up to par, here is my take on it...

A woman with SuperPowers, as defined by ME, is anyone who is RESPONSIBLE for anyone or anything and has to juggle multiple schedules to stay afloat.

This is a talent that only a woman can hold; sorry guys, multitasking at this speed is just not in your genes. A woman with SuperPowers can leap tall buildings in a single bound and still make sure homework is done, dinner is on the table, and her nails look halfway decent! It is that unstoppable zest for life, the overflowing energy, the Bing, Bang, Boom, that makes you AMAZING. It's a tough job, and only the strong do survive, but, as with any training regime, it only makes you stronger! So, with all that said, if you juggle a household schedule along with yours and sometimes feel like you have been hit by a Mack truck, this plan is just for YOU! This is your plan for energy, health, longevity, and some much deserved ME time. There are plenty of diet books, how-to books, and survival books out there and, although they fill the pages with some great information, they just don't have a clue as to how you can fit it all in and still have a smile on your face at the end of the day. We have become such a NOW society that everyone is trying to do everything all the time, and this works when we have the health and energy to keep up with ourselves; but if we don't, we just challenge ourselves past the point of no return.

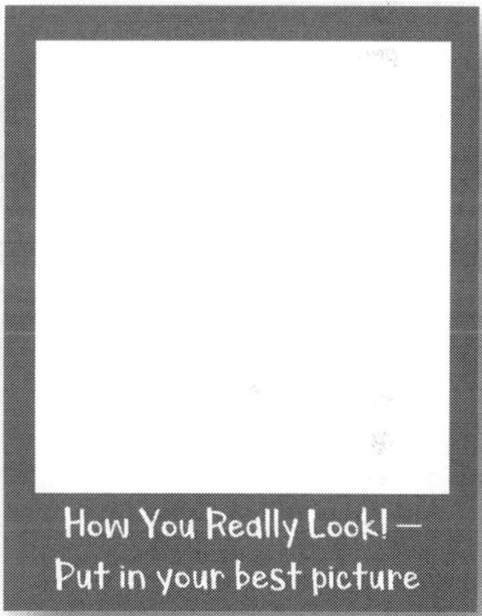

How You Really Look! — Put in your best picture

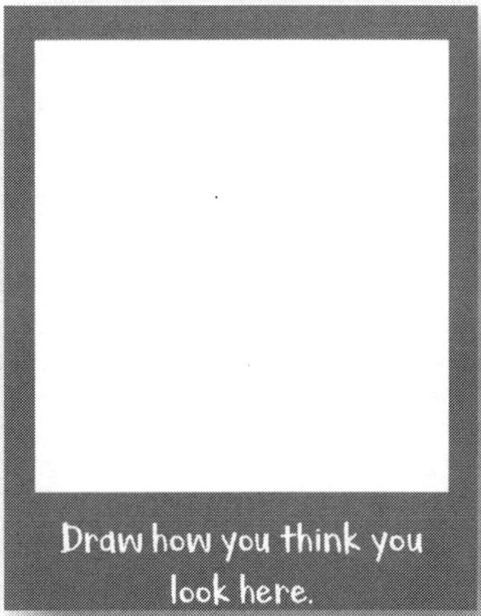

Draw how you think you look here.

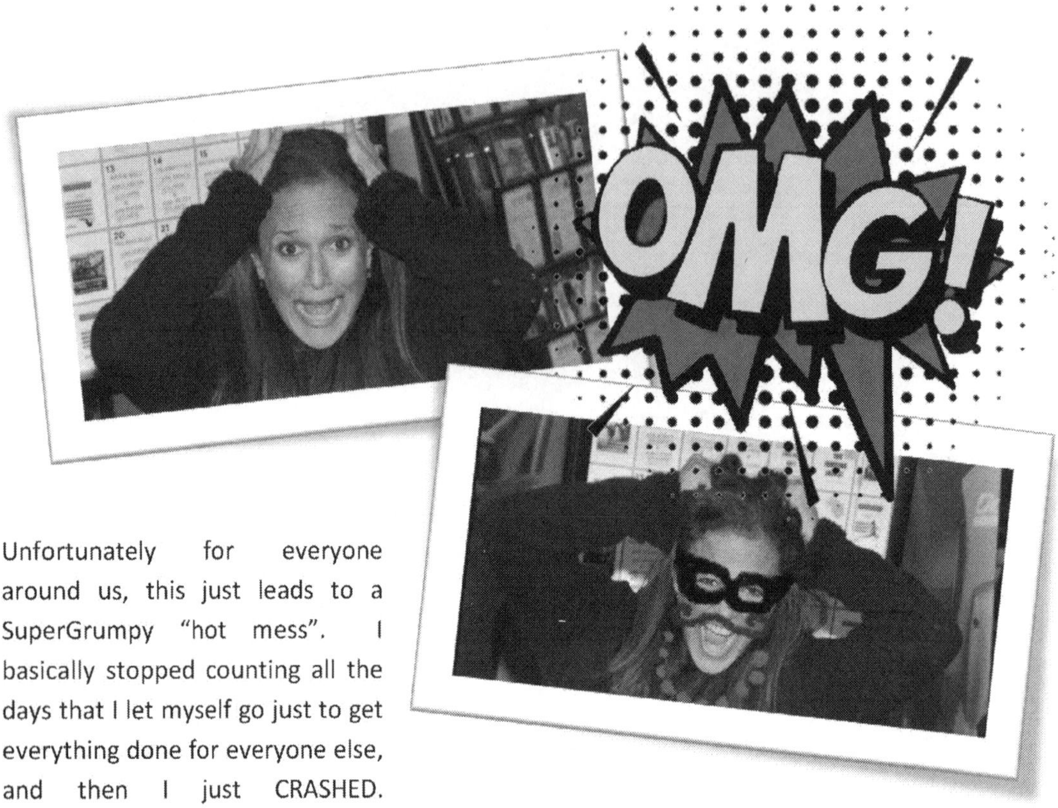

Unfortunately for everyone around us, this just leads to a SuperGrumpy "hot mess". I basically stopped counting all the days that I let myself go just to get everything done for everyone else, and then I just CRASHED.

I came to realize why they say, "It takes a village to run a family and a household." My SuperPowers started strong and fizzled out faster than ever. Some of you have "the gene" to get it all done, look great, and totally put your needs on the back burner, but that long run of SuperPowers will give up, if not this year then at some point. You and your health are the spark that keeps your SuperPowers SuperCharged for a lifetime!

I knew things had to change when eating a great lunch was in the car during traffic, and exercise was running errands before school pickup time. Exhaustion would set in at 2 p.m. and caffeine became my drug of choice; my SuperPowers were but a twinkle in my eye, actually I think they were hidden somewhere under the mounds of under-eye concealer. Here I am, the one who teaches people all about health and fitness, yet I am the one running on the hamster wheel without any means of stopping and hoping for my SuperPowers to reignite. Well, guess what?

There is a light at the end of the tunnel and it will make you shine like never before. All your SuperPowers need is 4 main ingredients. Are you listening? Hello, keep up because here are the secrets to fueling your Powers like never before...

The 4 Pillars of Health

Food & Nutrition • Exercise & Movement • Sleep & Relaxation

And my all-time favorite, the crème de la crème... Happiness and Joy!

SuperPowers need a balance of these for optimal performance, all 4 of them! Too much of one and not enough of the other will totally throw you off, but a balance of all will set your SuperPowers into full throttle, maximum output, and will last you until you say, "STOP!" Feeling great, motivated, and full of zest only empowers you to share the glory with your friends and family, WOW. But please don't get overwhelmed; I'm here to show you the easiest way possible to incorporate all of this into your busy schedule of activities and duties and show you that **IT CAN BE DONE**.

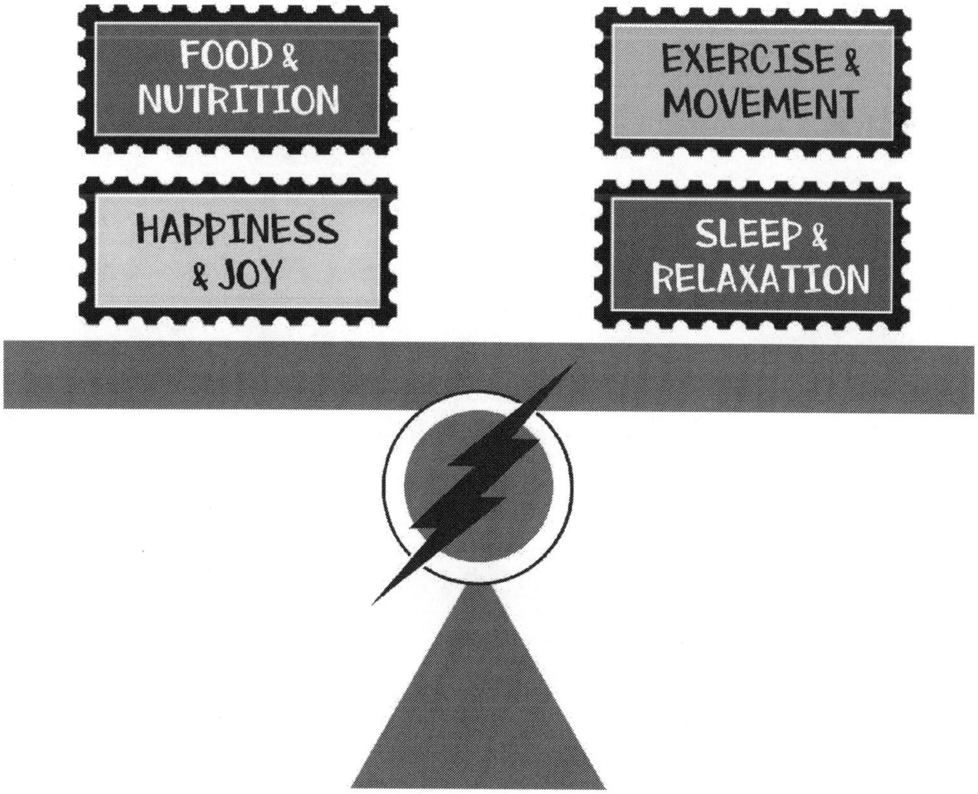

Juggling Family & Career

Health and fitness have been my love, my career, and my passion. They took me all over the world and gave me the opportunity to teach with some of the amazing minds of the wellness industry. The challenge came when I got married and had kids. OMG, no one told me the work involved, let alone the need to put oneself on the back burner, just to get by. Don't get me wrong, I love my family but I never imagined I would lead the road of so many of my clients. I remember "judging" my clients who just couldn't eat right or fit that one workout in—what was I thinking? OK, I was young, but I had no idea of the challenges that we can all face, let alone the intense impulse to place ourselves last, seriously, last! Considering I truly knew what was right and wrong, still I found myself right up there with the best. This has been one transformative journey. I can now better understand what all of those clients were going through, their emotions, exhaustion, and need for speed. With all this said I took a brief moment to reevaluate and create a system that works. It works for the craziest of lifestyles ... and trust me, I know!

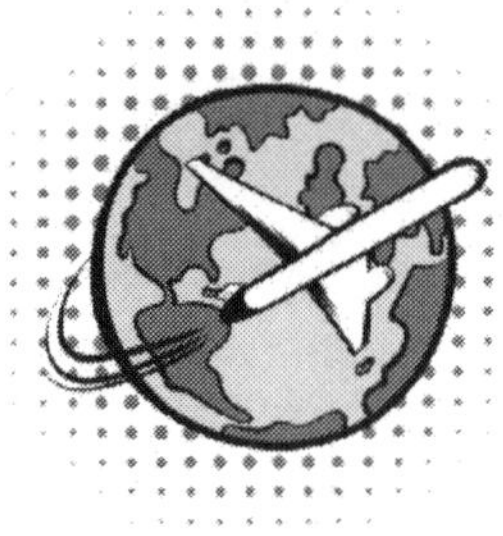

So there is no time to waste, let's get this show on the road and get you fueled up for some amazing days ahead!

THE WHO'S WHO OF FITNESS

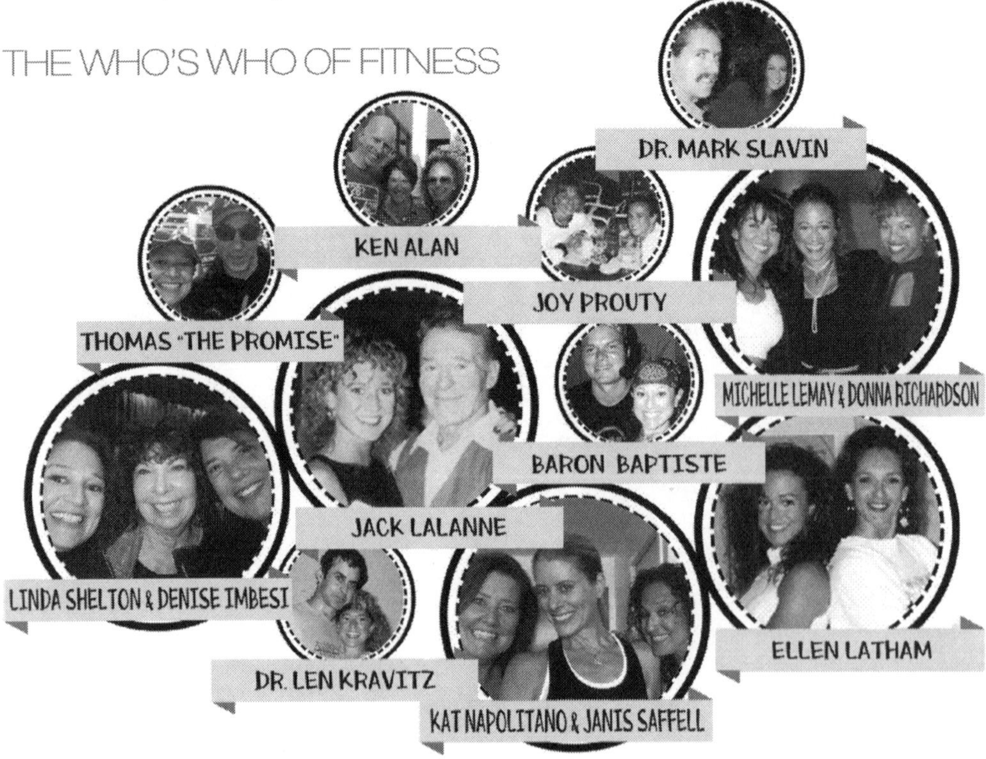

A SuperWoman's Ingredients for Maximum Power!

Life gets pretty funny; as I traveled on my own health journey and my extensive research into everything healthy it became clearer than ever that we are all just doing the best we can. Every gadget we buy, every machine we use comes with an in-depth instruction manual to get you out of the trickiest of situations, and they even have a "troubleshooting" section! Yet, here we are, simply left to our own devices. There is no instruction manual, we just try a little bit of this and a little bit of that and make up our own health. So if there is one thing I am gifting to you by the time you finish this book, it is the beginning of your personal instruction manual. Think of all of this as the outline, the essence of what you need to do. Then, depending on your schedule, motivations, taste buds, and more, you will fill in all of the necessary ingredients for it to fit into your life, smooth as silk!

Health is an amazing thing, but unfortunately there is no one thing that encompasses complete health. Only a balanced approach will lead to a strong foundation of great health and longevity deserved by all SuperWomen alike. As I mentioned before, the primary ingredients that create a strong foundation for our health are the following:

Food and Nutrition, here comes your SuperPower Fuel Plan. Any SuperWoman knows how important it is to feel energized and to think clearly with all of those thoughts rattling through our brains. The right food choices can enhance our energy, recuperation, and so much more. No matter how you look at it, we are the pack leader and as that amazing figurehead we must shine at all times and our food is that one thing that will speed up our recuperation and keep us level-headed for the trenches!

Next up, **Exercise and Movement**, this is where your SuperPower Training Regime will show its true colors. Not to fret, by no means am I sending you to the gym for hours, this is doable... I promise. Then you can't forget **Sleep and Relaxation**, here you have the chance to reignite your energy, take a well-deserved "time out", and recharge your battery for more zest in Life!

And of course, last but not nearly least, we have to be **HAPPY**; we need to charge up our happiness cells to their very max. We need to laugh like no one is watching, and even if they are we should enjoy it like never before.

Please don't let any of this overwhelm you, I have been through it all and I am here to tell you that *you got this*. Getting yourself to balance these 4 pillars is going to make you feel so amazing that your newly acquired habits will just take over. The changes will be small and simple, but the rewards will make it so very worth it.

Your SuperPowers
deserve the very best!

NUTRITION. EXERCISE. SLEEP. HAPPINESS.

SELFIE

PLACE YOUR BEST SELFIE HERE

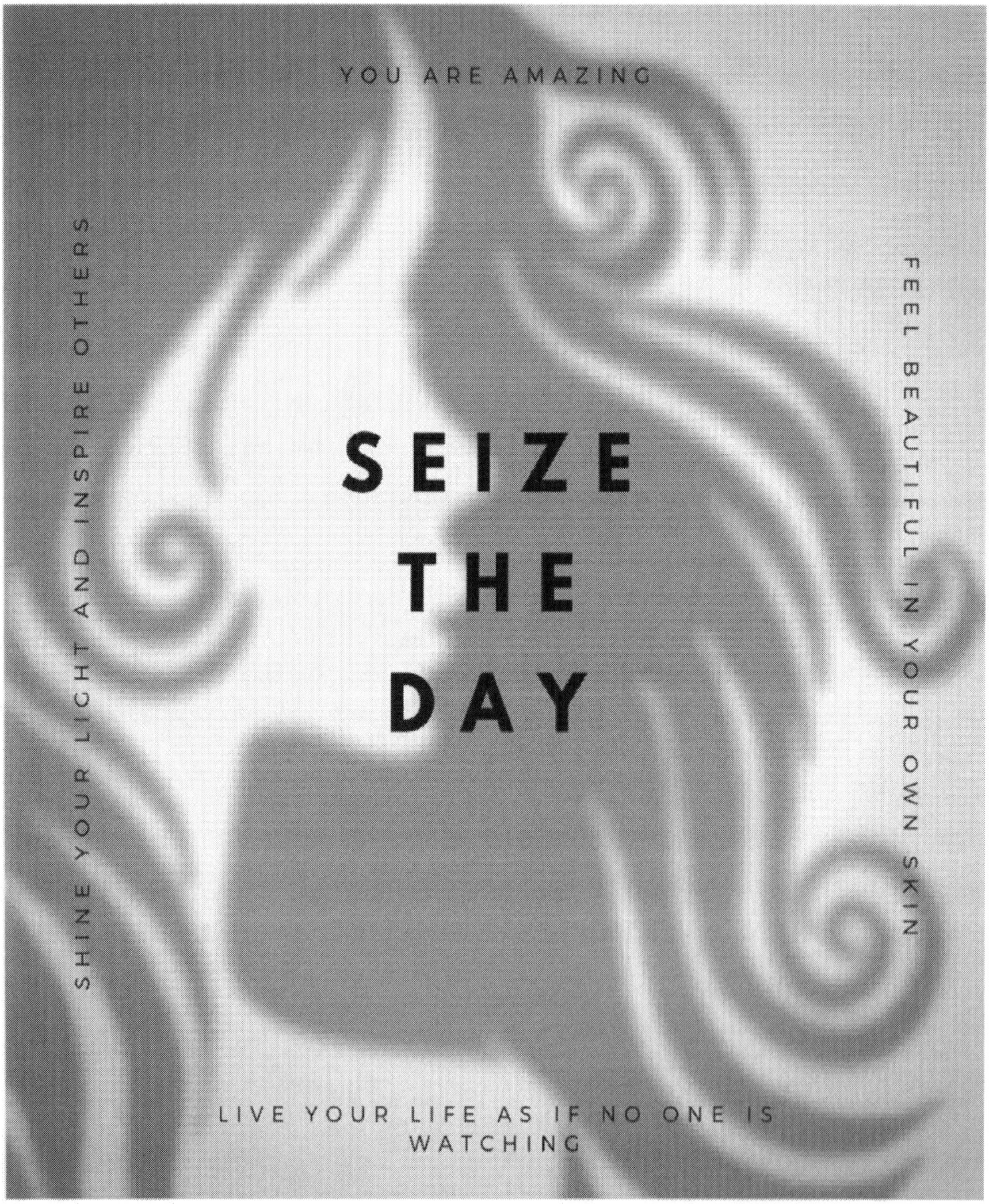

"The right fuel ignites an unstoppable force in any amazing machine, so just imagine what it will do for you!"

-with Love,

Adita Lang♡

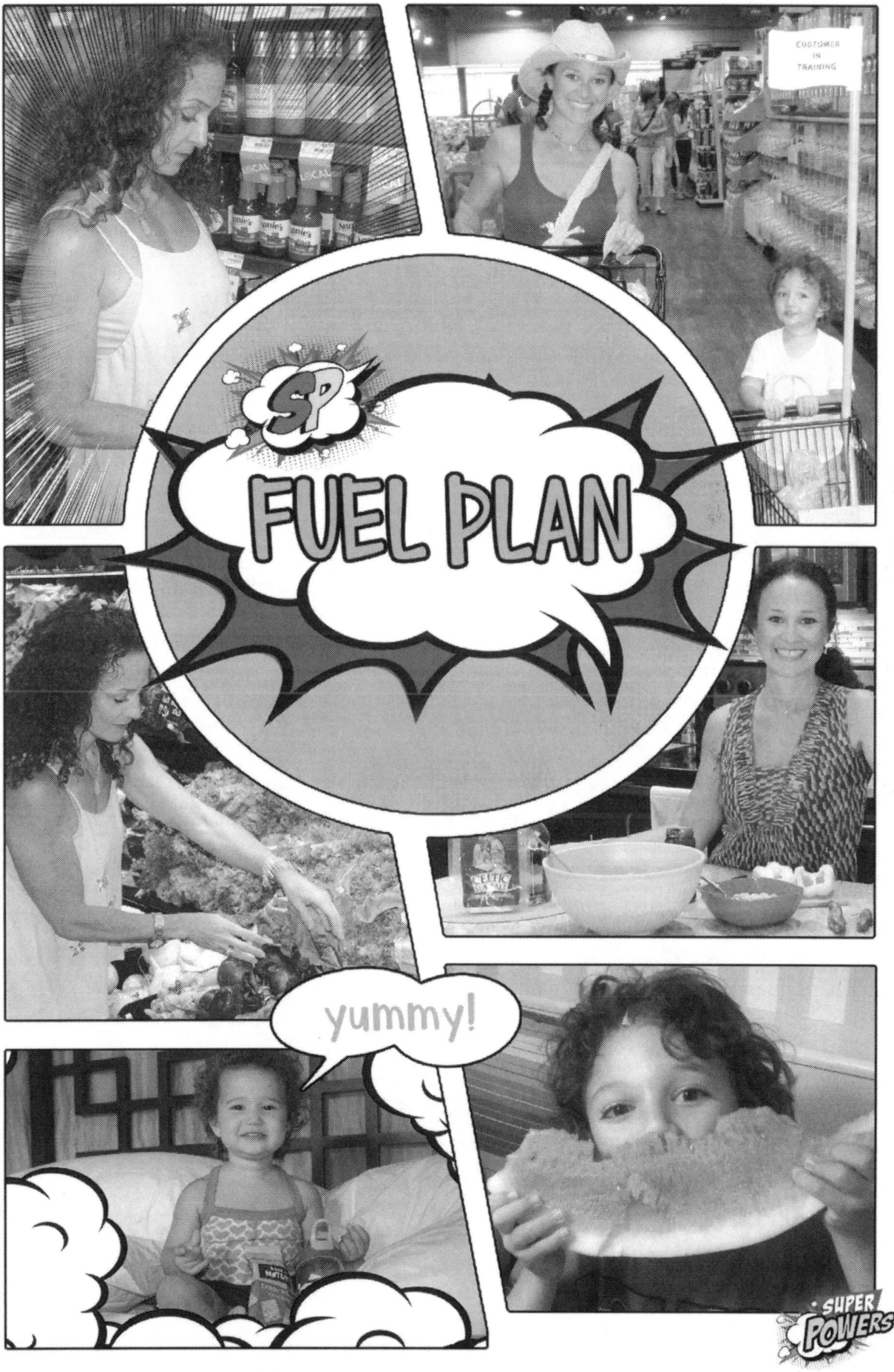
CUSTOMER
IN
TRAINING
SP
FUEL PLAN
yummy!
SUPER
POWERS

SuperPower Fuel Plan

OK, pay attention, this is so much easier than most people think, actually I think most of my girlfriends tend to overthink this and that begins the cyclone of terror. Food is fuel; that is the bottom line. If you served up a Big Mac and cheese to a Maserati you would not get very far, well girl, the same happens to you! Too many people have sugarcoated this life thing; I am here to tell you as it is. We were all raised thinking that food was social, enjoyable, fun, IT'S NOT! It can be enjoyable as long as it is the *Joy of Cooking*, it is meant to SuperCharge your body and that is about it.

I always knew that the right foods were important; now, whether I lived by that or not is a totally different thing. Honestly, I don't think it really hit me until I was pregnant with my first child. I ate better than most but still loved my treats and my Diet Cokes. When I was pregnant with Nash, a dear friend said that I was "growing a baby from scratch," WOW! This took me to a whole new light as it came to my foods, I had no intention of growing a Diet Coke baby, my baby was going to be filled with spinach and pasture fed eggs! Then, not to mention that my pelvic floor was heading downhill and my exercise regime came to a full halt. I was left with two choices: gorge my way to "baby fat" or eat in such a manner that I was growing the next SuperHero for Marvel comics. As you can guess, I chose the SuperHero and the changes I made, as subtle as they were, changed my body even better than my past 20 hour a week of fitness ever did. I came to have a new respect for foods and the nutritional density that they can provide. I had preached it for years but when I was left without my workouts and with food as my only friend, I found a new meaning to health, energy, and mental clarity that I had never known.

What is Nutrition? Nutrition is the process of "powering up" your body for everything your day has to offer. It's about breaking down foods so that you can use what you need, how you need it, and never have to beg, borrow or steal from other parts of your body just to get your engines started. Your body needs certain nutrients and your mind needs others, so how can you expect to be energized, cheery, and in 12 different places at once unless you have the right quality fuel to make this happen? Studies show that people committed to an exercise program tend to eat well and are more mentally alert; well, these studies didn't take into account true SuperPowers, the kind that keep you moving from here to there for hours without giving thought to healthy food or even sitting down to eat. Life can get carried away, but now it's time to change those habits and to create new ones that will be your true lifelong friends!

Nutrition 101

For abundant energy, lean muscles, and great health we need a few things – Carbohydrates, Proteins, Fats, Enzymes, Vitamins, Minerals, and Water. But not all of these from your local supermarket are created equal.

Your body builds muscle, promotes health, strengthens your immune system, amps up your battery, and clears your mind all with the right quality and combinations of foods. So here are the nuts and bolts so you can start to see the light.

Carbohydrates – These guys give us immediate energy, fuel our brain, and zap our muscles for performance. They come in two varieties...

SIMPLE

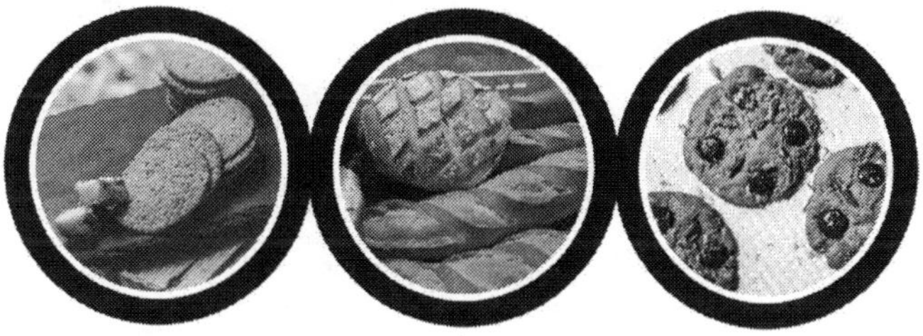

Simple – Unfortunately these are the ones we crave; they make us fat, yet in a happy sort of a way. These primarily come from processed foods; yup, those foods that have been manufactured in some shape or form. They are easy to use and consume; they can give us a lot of energy but at a terrible cost to the hips and thighs. These include sugar, flour, processed cereals, cookies, cupcakes and so much more. Sugar, flour, dairy, and alcohol all, pretty much, metabolize as a sugar and our bodies love to store them. For some strange reason our brain makes us feel OHHH SOOOO comforted as soon as we eat one, or two, or even three. Now, one thing to remember is that most of these things also include corn syrup or high fructose corn syrup and these guys are EVIL. Yes, they are addictive and they can easily spike your bad cholesterol and your body fat. Did you know that some soda manufacturers make their sodas with high fructose corn syrup solely for Americans? On the other hand Europeans will not stand for it! Oh ya, they have us hooked and they work very hard at keeping it that way, hmmm.

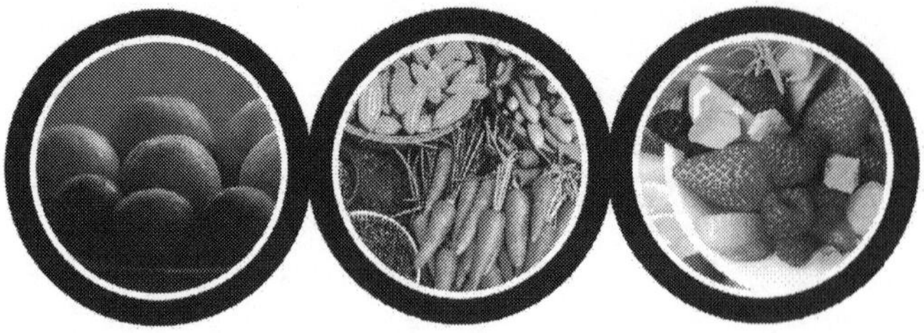

COMPLEX

Complex – Now this is the good stuff. It gives us a steadier stream of SuperPower Energy because it is packed with vitamins, minerals, and fiber. These include fruits and vegetables and unprocessed grains. The dietary fiber helps to clean up the body of nasty toxins and is a powerhouse of energy to help us maximize our day. These guys work best when minimally processed. Combined with the right kind of fat and proteins, complex carbohydrates can give you tons of energy no matter how out of hand your schedule becomes—they are your friends.

PROTEINS

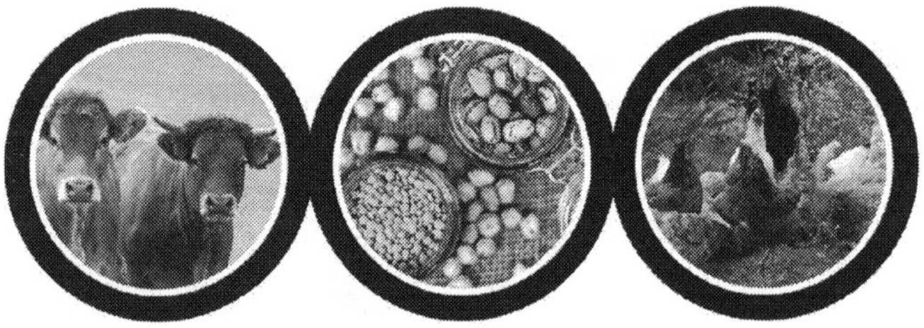

Proteins – Muscles need these to be big and strong and our body uses these for repair and to place that wonderful energy from complex carbohydrates on cruise control. It's an important part of being lean and sexy. Protein takes longer to break down and digest so it actually helps us have energy and feel fuller for a longer period of time when combined with good quality carbohydrates and quality fats.

They include chicken, fish, meat, eggs, legumes, grains, leafy greens, seeds, and nuts. Probably the most important thing to understand is that proteins are like a computer code and if they are missing a piece of the puzzle we don't get the full benefit. With this said, beans are wonderful but they are not complete so you need to combine these with either grains or seeds to finish off the code (i.e. beans and rice, garbanzos and tahini for hummus, etc.). Vegetarians need to be aware of this. People who don't eat meat, fish, poultry or eggs need to eat a variety of foods containing protein each day in order to get all the amino acids needed to make a complete protein.

Proteins are considered the building blocks of the body, every cell in the human body contains protein and it helps to build and repair cells, as well as muscle tissue. At least 10,000 different proteins make you what you are with your unique framework of strength, health, and overall longevity.

So how much protein do you need?

Let's not get crazy about this, just try to include a good quality protein with every meal and snack and you will be good to go! Your goal is about 40% of each of your meals and snacks, but different things in our day can change that. A few examples are...

Daily Activity Level – A lot of exercise would require a higher proportion of carbohydrates for immediate energy, proteins to keep that energy going for a while and for muscular repair, and quality fats for extended energy—kind of like a reserve.

How Much Protein, Carbohydrates, and Fats do we need with each meal or snack?

Daily Food Planning – If you have a full day and way too much time between meals, you would increase your protein and fat proportion so that the calories you eat would last longer in your system and keep you fuller. This is imperative so that the minute you get a chance to sit and recover you don't eat everything in sight! A good example of a breakfast that needs to last for as many hours as possible is an omelet with veggies and a side of fruit; when you look at the proportions there should be more protein from the eggs, a smaller amount of carbs from the veggies and fruit, and a small amount of fat from the olive oil. This will keep you satiated for hours.

For High Stress or Illness – High quality, nutritionally dense proteins would need to be amped up to keep you on an even keel all day long and to help you recover at your very best.

How long should these keep you full for?

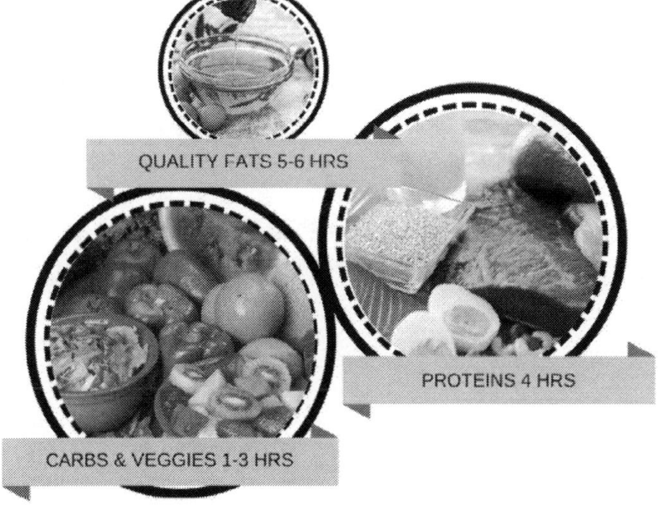

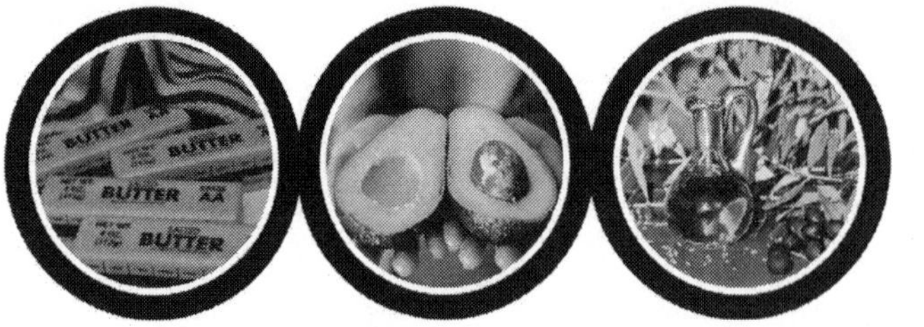

FATS

Fats – Don't be fooled, these guys are far from being your #1 enemy! We need fat; fat protects our organs, gives us soft skin and hair, and provides us with energy when all of our other calories have run out. Yup, think of these guys as your "battery backup", the challenge is choosing the right stuff to do the job. For your purposes, there are two forms of fat—good and bad. Crazily enough, saturated fat can also be good and bad. Most people think of it as the bad stuff; it can be cut off of meat and is a thicker, denser substance as in lard. It is the place where all toxins are stored and become concentrated. But here is the catch, good quality, as in 100% grass fed butter or meat, can actually be good for you, again it's ALL about quality! On the other hand, bad saturated fats have nothing good about them other than adding fat to your waistline and packing it in your arteries. Mono-unsaturated is the good stuff, it is more liquid in nature, brings in several essential nutrients, and helps to protect our internal organs and acts as a lubricant for the body. These fats include cold-pressed/unrefined olive oil, coconut oil, and flaxseed oil. Fat can also help to provide sustained energy when combined with quality protein and carbohydrates.

Here's a little more to really clear up all of this "fat confusion". Let's look at the so-called bad and then good so you can compare and come up with your own opinion.

Saturated fat – Yuck (but only sometimes), this is the sticky stuff that causes your cholesterol levels to rise and increases your chances of cardiovascular disease. It is the solid type of fat that comes from animal sources, such as red meat, poultry and full-fat dairy products. Here is where your BAD low-density lipoprotein (LDL) cholesterol levels go up and your health goes down, it's even been linked to type 2 diabetes. But there is a flip side, according to the *British Medical Journal*, *Annals of Internal Medicine*, the Weston Price Foundation and several others who have been involved in the research studies on saturated fat, quality saturated fat has several beneficial factors for human health, WHAT? We are more at risk from processed vegetable oils than we are of a stick of grass fed butter. Once again the main key here is all on the quality of our choices (have I emphasized "quality" enough?), so here's the skinny (no pun intended):

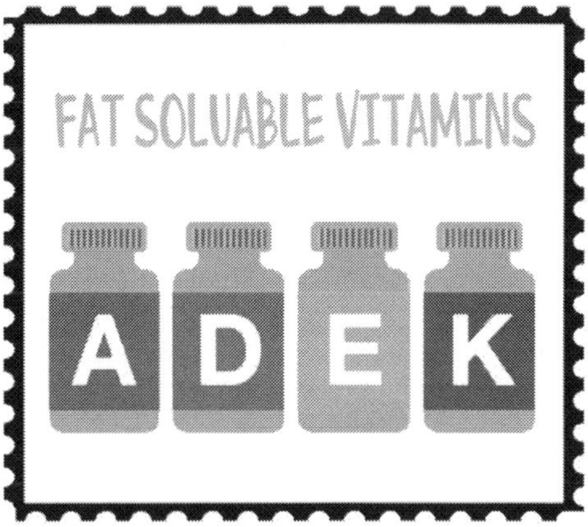

✱ Vitamins A, D, E, and K are actually found in saturated fat and can only be absorbed in the body with the use of fat. You'll learn more about these guys in the pages that follow, but just remember that we need these vitamins badly!

✱ Saturated fats are a main initiator for the manufacturing of both testosterone and estrogen, so if you really want to keep your wits sharp, don't leave home without them!

✱ Saturated fats are a critical component of our nervous system and ensure the proper function of the nerves.

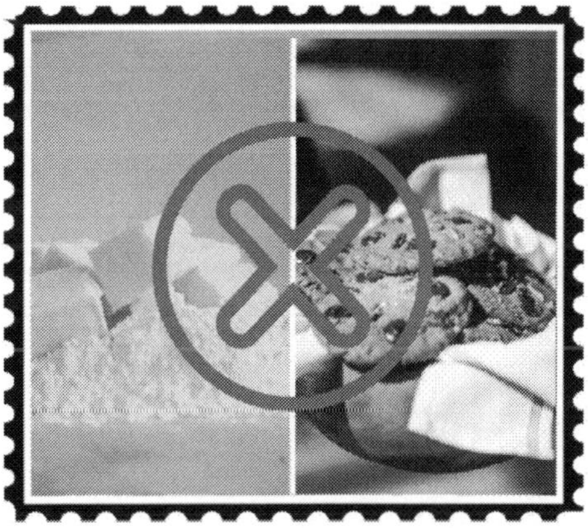

✱ Saturated fats help to reduce inflammation as long as they are consumed away from processed carbohydrates. This is important to understand because when you combine saturated fats with flour and sugar, as in some amazing butter and sugar cookies, they produce inflammation in the body. This is what made them so bad in the first place. The combination created an unhealthy response in the body. Consuming quality saturated fats away from flour and sugar actually reduces inflammation and provides the body with additional benefits.

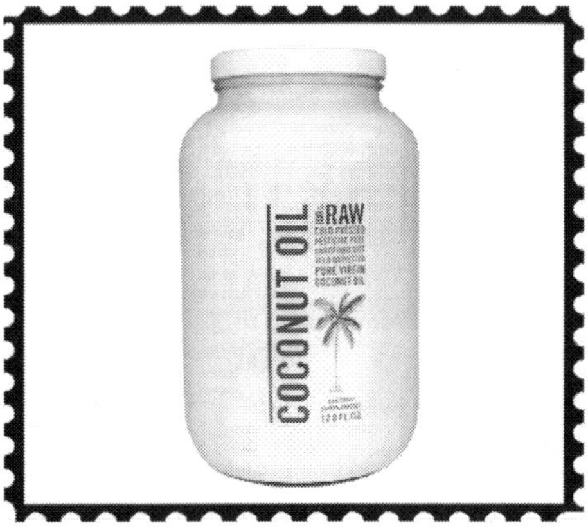

✱ The saturated fat components from both grass fed butter and coconut oil actually strengthen the immune system and assist in cellular communication throughout the body. This in turn helps with cancer and several other health challenges that our SuperPower bodies can live without.

Trans fat – This is the icky stuff! There is an itty bitty teeny tiny bit that comes naturally in some of our foods but the majority is man-made, manufactured, yuck! They call it partial hydrogenation, it's a fancy term that means they modified it, manufactured it, and processed it enough to make our lives easier; it heats up quicker, stores in the pantry for years to come and can increase unhealthy LDL cholesterol and lower healthy high-density lipoprotein (HDL) cholesterol. Your risk of cardiovascular disease goes up and your health tumbles, but it's easier to use, ya right. Just like its saturated fat counterpart, it is solid at room temperature but does the body NO GOOD.

Here's the stuff that has always been highlighted as GOOD.
It's simply about "how" they are used that
really shows their true potential:

Monounsaturated fat – This type of fat is found in a variety of foods and oils naturally. Studies show that eating foods rich in monounsaturated fats (MUFAs) improves blood cholesterol levels, which decreases your risk of heart disease, now that's a plus! Research also shows that type 2 diabetes receives great gains with benefits in insulin levels and blood sugar control. (Keep in mind that fat will slow down the spike of sugar during digestion, this is why it aids in blood sugar control)

Polyunsaturated fat – This wonderful fat is found mostly in plant-based foods and oils and provides all of the same benefits as its buddy, monounsaturated fat.

Omega-3 fatty acid – Here's a type of polyunsaturated fat that is made up of mainly omega-3 fatty acids and is quite beneficial to your heart. Omega-3, found in some types of fatty fish and some foods, appears to decrease the risk of coronary artery disease, protect against irregular heartbeats, lower blood pressure levels, and ... FEED THE BRAIN! Gotta love that! The body prefers the fish-based omega, but, hey, you still can't go wrong with plant sources either, so just get it in there and stop forgetting where you placed your keys!

Foods made up mostly of monounsaturated and polyunsaturated fats are liquid at room temperature, such as olive oil. Fish high in omega-3 fatty acids include salmon, tuna, trout, mackerel, sardines and herring, but watch out for that nasty mercury and plastics found in some fish, you have to be choosy. Plant sources of omega-3 fatty acids include flaxseeds (ground and oil) and raw nuts and seeds (walnuts, cashews, almonds, etc., and their raw nut butter counterparts, also all the raw seeds like chia, hemp and sunflower).

Cholesterol – GOOD or BAD, should we flip a coin?
Here is the true "ugly" of all fat issues we have—

HDL is GOOD and LDL is BAD.

Most cholesterol is produced in the body as a defense mechanism against arterial "scrapes"; yes you heard it right, some foods such as corn syrup and high fructose corn syrup are challenging to break down during the digestive process. They require so much effort that arteries are slightly damaged, scratched up or just wounded so the body produces cholesterol to repair and resurface the area. With this said, foods only provoke your body to produce cholesterol, cholesterol from foods does not typically "stick" to your arteries during digestion. There are some people who were passed on some funky genes and they form excess cholesterol with and without these provoking foods, if you are one of these people you will always have cholesterol issues ideally you keep it monitored by your doctor and keep it high in HDL!

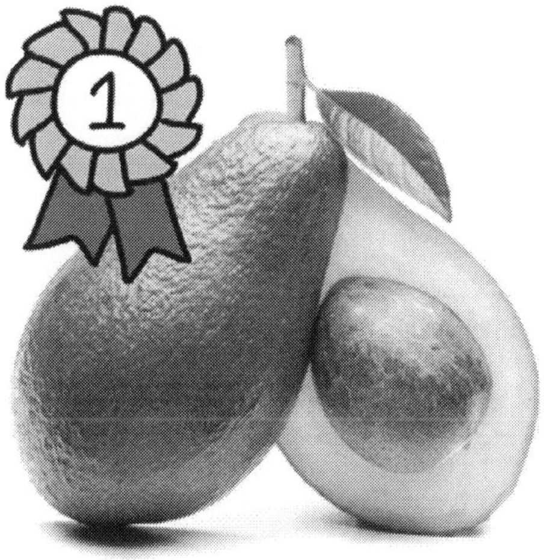

So you do have some bad stuff out there, but the majority is pretty good. There are still so many other wonderful things that quality fat can do for us. As with all foods, nutritional density is the key; choose fats that provide you with added nutrients and the body will reap the benefits. Processed fats and oils are lacking enzymes and have been altered from their natural state. Fats that are naturally derived from a food source with little to no processing can provide us with an array of benefits. Our top choices are: cold pressed un-refined coconut oil, cold pressed un-refined olive oil, organic grass fed butter*, organic grass fed ghee, organic grass fed meats, bone broth, cold pressed un-refined organic nut oils, avocados, raw nuts, and organic/pasture fed eggs—you simply have to choose the best of the best because your body WILL NOT settle for less!

SUPERPOWER favorite ... The winner is avocado!

*I emphasize "organic grass fed" because this actually changes the nutritional density of the butter or meat. When a cow is fed a processed meal, the nutrient content of that cow changes, pesticide residue increases, and the way we digest and utilize the food changes as well. This leaves us with meat that increases our LDL and provides little if any quality nutrition.

Oh boy, hold the presses, one more valuable tidbit about fat, if you're hooked on caffeine because it is the only way to have a civilized conversation first thing in the morning then you need this tidbit! Here it is, don't be scared, this truly is not gross, just read this with an open mind. Are you ready? Add a teaspoon or so of coconut oil to your coffee or tea. This will slow down the caffeine from entering your system, giving you the "high" for a longer period of time without stressing out your system and giving you that sudden drop of energy. See, that wasn't so bad and coconut oil has sooo much to give—it helps regulate your hormones, is great for skin and nails, great for your gums, it even helps keep your teeth white while you drink your tea and coffee ... who knew!

As you can see, everything seems to work together and it all depends on the excellence of your food choices. We spend numerous hours choosing just the right handbag, not to mention the right outfit and shoes. Starting today, I want you to put that much attention and value on the foods you eat. Your stunning appearance is not simply from your makeup and cool threads, it has to do with the health inside you shining outward and making you glow like never before. Let me tell you, by the time you add in just a few changes to your day, you will look stunning in your grubbiest clothes!

Now, as I mentioned earlier, nothing works alone, so here are the valuable parts of all foods that give us that "glowing shine".

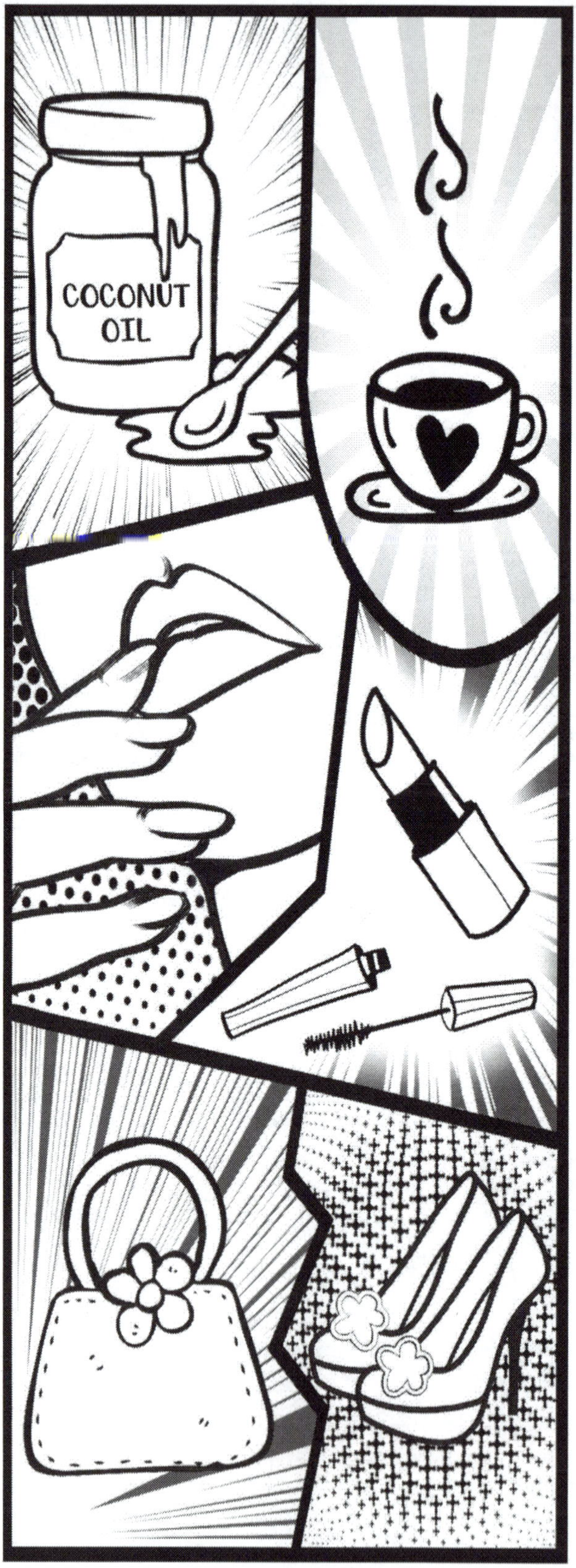

Feel free to color me in!

vitamins

These are the heavy hitters that perform every internal action that is necessary to make you jam! They are a non-caloric substance that can be classified as water soluble or fat soluble. Water soluble vitamins (such as B and C) are absorbed directly into the blood stream. Fat soluble are the ones I mentioned earlier, they are stored in the fatty tissue of the body, so if you're not eating fat you are totally missing out on these guys (such as A, D, E and K). But here is the catch, although it might seem easier to take these from a bottle, the body really doesn't recognize the man-made, manufactured, knock-offs that you find in the store. Your body wants FOODS, it wants to get its nutrients from FOODS, so don't get crazy and buy all this bottled stuff, save your money and spend it on fresh organics instead.

Top Vitamin Picks and their Benefits

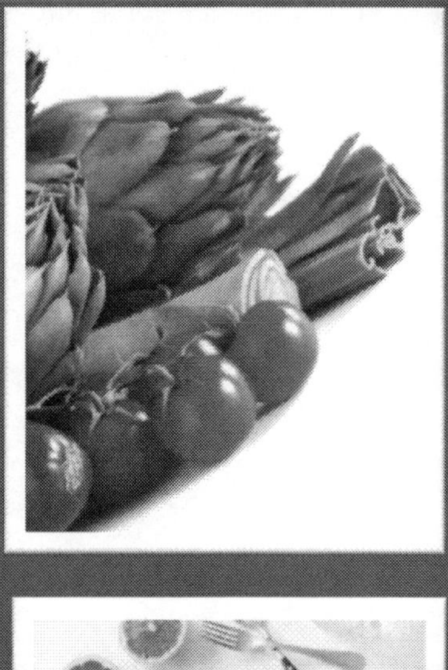

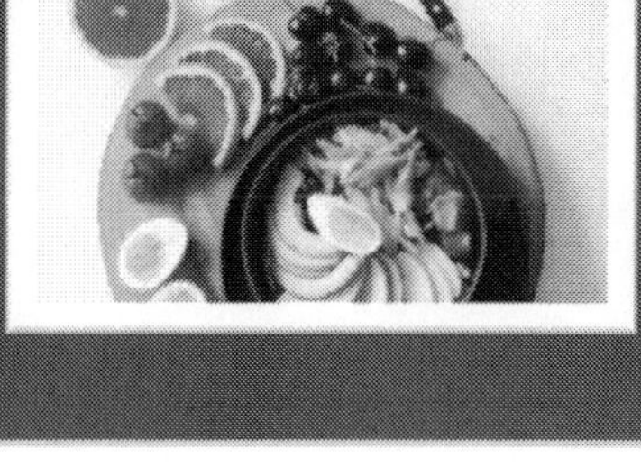

Vitamin A	Keeps the skin supple and the eyesight sharp.
Vitamin B	Breaks down those cookies with ease and cranks up your SuperPower energy centers.
Vitamin C	Boosts your immune system and makes sure everything is working in top gear and repairs better than ever.
Vitamin D	Makes bones strong and ready for any adventure you put your sights on, and this one is free. Just 10-15 minutes of sun should do the trick.
Vitamin E	This one gives you soft skin, strong muscles, and is the key ingredient to all repair.
Vitamin K	Maintains your blood working just the right way for you.

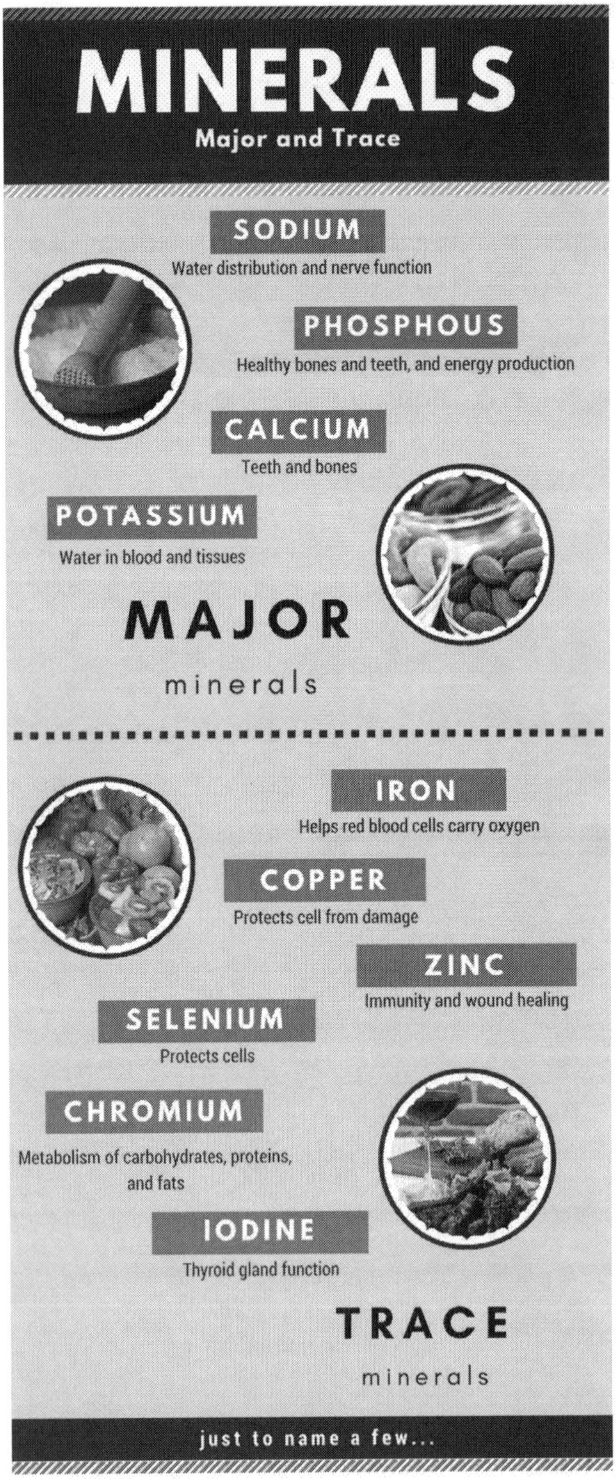

Minerals – Although you don't hear that much about them, they are just as important. They, too, are found in your foods and come to you in just the right amounts as long as you're eating a healthy diet. We have major minerals (macro minerals) and trace minerals (micro minerals). Both of these are equally important and have specific job duties for the body's internal processes, yet trace minerals are typically needed in smaller quantities than major minerals. They are both naturally occurring but inorganic in nature. The table shows some of my top pics and the benefits they produce.

OK are you ready? Here is The Secret Element of Food Success, the Mecca of it all, the one thing that assures you that you are receiving and absorbing everything your foods promised you…

Are you curious? Well, I gave you vitamins and minerals, but there is still one missing piece of the puzzle—the one thing no one really talks about, and the one thing that truly makes all the difference in the world. Our body is designed to optimally function on quality fuel that provides vitamins, minerals and...Enzymes. Enzymes are like a computer code that tells our body specifically what to do with everything we eat, each nutrient, fat, and crumb; the key is that enzymes only survive in raw, unprocessed foods. For example: the enzymes of an apple will tell the body what to do with the vitamins, minerals, and fiber, and anything extra gets tossed from there. Enzymes are the magic compound of RAW foods! They are the ones that work with the body to do the following:

- They are in high demand for every chemical reaction of the body
- They are connected to every working organ of the body and run life's processes (including weight loss!)
- Who do you think keeps the body clean? It's not a typical shower but they assist the body with detoxification and cleansing
- They break down all of your foods and distribute the nutrients throughout the body
- They are the SuperHeroes of the digestive process
- But they are not invincible, they are easily destroyed with heat (<105 degrees), as in cooking, and are totally non-existent in processed and manufactured foods

Enzymes come in several varieties with numerous jobs throughout the body. Digestive enzymes are designed to help break down foods and assist the body's distribution system for the nutrients, fiber, and the disposal of any unnecessary parts. In other words, food that is raw or has been heated at or below 105 degrees provides the body with an array of digestive enzymes that tell the body how to use and organize all of the great things found in the foods you are eating. Unfortunately, heat and processing kill off these valuable SuperHeroes, making it harder for the body to break down and organize all of the great things found in foods and making it much easier to store everything (even the good stuff) as fat!

We do store excess digestive enzymes and we can use them to break down cooked foods; the challenge arises when we don't eat enough raw foods to replenish our stores. When we run out of enzymes, our bodies easily become exhausted processing all of the foods. This, in turn leads to a lazy system and a metabolism that wants to go on strike. Yup, when you don't have enough digestive enzymes your body takes the "easy way out" and stores it all in the fat cells, leaving us with fewer nutrients and larger fat reserves. The key to staying lean and creating a digestive machine is to eat a lot of raw food choices throughout the day or to combine raw with cooked so that you are always on the straight track of lean and energized!

Here are a few things to remember when your enzymes are down and out:

1. Foods can be easily stored as fat, UGH!

2. Nutrients are stolen from body reserves for digestion.

It is all pretty simple, focus on quality foods in their natural, unprocessed state, and leave that calorie counting to some chump who has the time. You deserve all of the wonderful benefits of food and you shouldn't have to work that hard at it, so let's check out a few more things that can set us on the right path for good!

Last but not least, this one might not be your favorite but it sure does give you everything and more...
Water – This is the major element for all of the workings of the human body. Without water all of that cardio you torture yourself with only leads to muscle breakdown instead of major fat disposal. Water is a critical element of the body, and great hydration is a must for the body to function at 100%. Up to 75% of the body's weight is made up of water. Most of the water is found within the cells of the body and here is where it distributes all of our wonderful nutrients. Water is responsible for "de-gunking" our insides, removing any metabolic by-products and toxins that are tarnishing our system. Water works side by side with the liver to break down fat efficiently through cardiovascular training and works directly in the muscle to assist muscular contraction for strength gain. A decrease in water leads to dehydration and for any woman that can mean anything from fatigue to muscle breakdown, and even a "slow down" in the fat burning process.

We are all very unique so our demands on water are very specific to our size, activity level, and the lean muscle mass that we hold so dear. The average individual should follow this formula as a guide:

- A minimum of 8 glasses of H2O a day
- Add 2 more glasses of H20 every time you drink something with caffeine or alcohol
- Double check how well you're doing by checking out the color of your urine (clear is optimal)

Since our bodies are so frickin smart we get some signals that we really should pay attention to. When the body is short on fluids it sends out that feeling of thirst; if you don't pay attention it sends out the next alarm of hunger. Hunger can just be thirst in a funky costume, the body will send out this signal in hopes of extracting fluids from the food. You may not be hungry, you may have eaten way too many calories at an earlier time, but your body is resorting to this cheap trick just to get a glass of water. Caffeine, alcohol and certain medications can also contribute to dehydration and this incredible lack of water. These should be kept to a minimum, but if you really need that cup of joe or the kids have driven you to drink, then add in a few more glasses of water to help counterbalance the effects.

Now, with that all said, there is one great thing that can substitute for water—raw coconut water. Here's a wonderful return on your investment, coconut water replaces the fluids and minerals that the body loses during physical activities and SuperPower endeavors. Even the United Nations Food and Agriculture Organization (FAO) attested to the benefits of drinking coconut water when it fought for a patent in 2000 to market coconut water as the next big sports drinks.

Basically, coconut water is like natural Gatorade®. It contains water, simple carbohydrates (or sugar), naturally occurring enzymes, and electrolytes (or minerals). Compared to a sports drink made with refined sugars, artificial flavoring, synthetically derived nutrients and food coloring, I'd say coconut water represents a solid upgrade. To top that off, coconut water keeps our digestion at its best, helps fend off a nasty cold, and gives your skin everything it needs to shine.

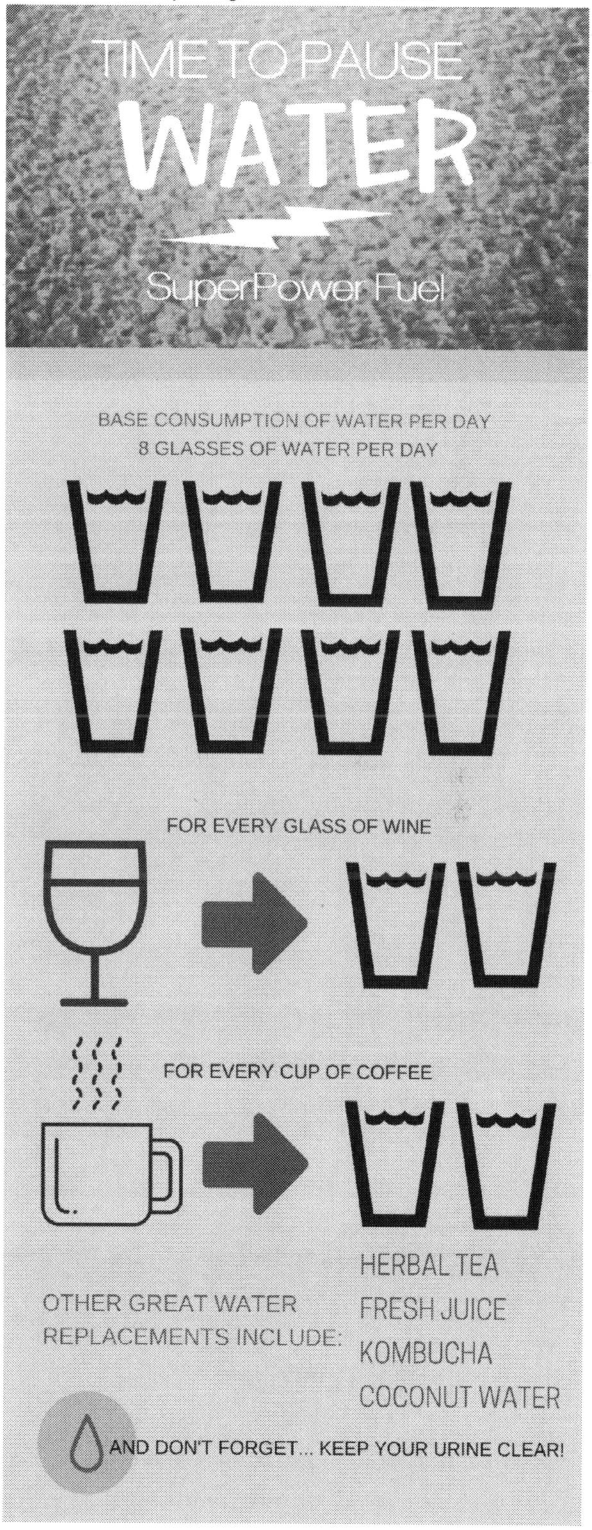

How Does This All Come Together?

I have just given you my "Nutrition 101"; this is the essence of all human function as it applies to food. Proper digestion begins the moment we put food or liquids into our mouth. Digestive enzymes begin to break down the food into its own unique components and water distributes them throughout the body to the areas that need them the most. This absorption of nutrients gives us the energy to conquer our day, kick some major booty, and provides us the strength for a healthy body free from illness and disease. Everything we consume has nutritional value, some more than others, this helps to enhance the health of our bodies. As a society we have been programmed to eat for depression, a party or simply for fun. Our bodies are SuperSmart and if they get everything they need, they shine, they give us that power to leap tall buildings in a single bound, and they give us the strength to make each day better than the last. Many of us make food choices that lack the nutrients we need, so our bodies scream out, "I'm Hungry, FEED ME!" and we keep eating until that one vitamin we are craving is located. Your body is like a fine-tuned automobile and if you fill it with high quality premium fuel and take good care of it, it will perform like never before. On the other hand, if you fill it with low grade fuel and skip the tune-up here and there, it will take you down; you will feel trampled on by something you never saw coming!

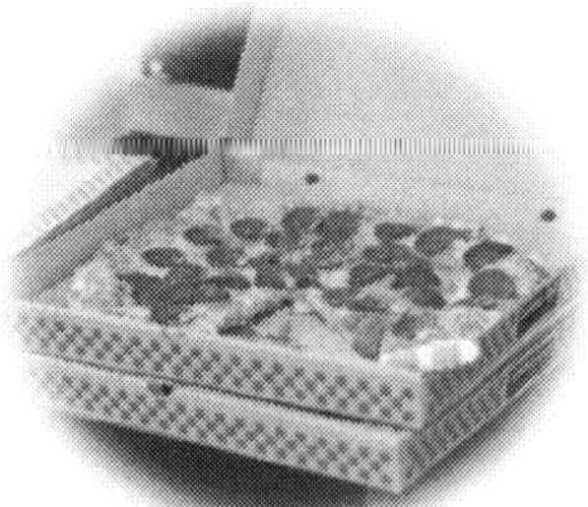

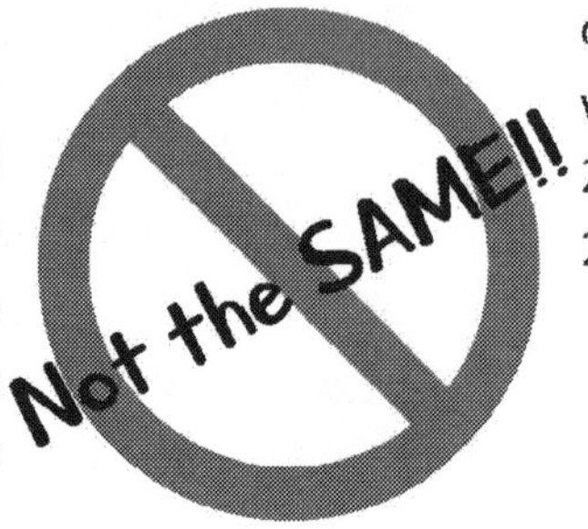

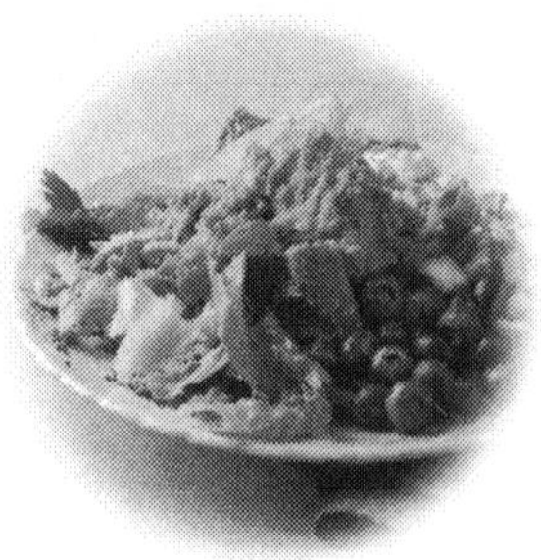

You are a woman with SuperPowers, not a force to be reckoned with! Your primary power source comes from your foods; you want nutritionally dense foods that reward your body with good health. Remember that 200 calories of pizza is not equal to 200 calories of vegetables and fish.

You may be providing your body with the caloric energy it needs, but the lack of nutrients will make the body desire more food until its nutritional needs have been met. Once your body is fulfilled with high quality foods, its need and desire for lower quality foods will dissipate and you will charge forward stronger than ever.

Things to Know

Before we choose the right foods for your plan, *Let's debunk some typical misconceptions and more!*

Every SuperPowered woman I know started on this journey with the very best of intentions, they had plans of grandeur to feed their families and themselves the very best; they had visions of that beautiful apron and these amazing, picture perfect meals at every dinner. And then reality set in and time became of the essence, but the sad part is that food manufacturers took note of these weaknesses and sabotaged us like never before. They know we don't have the time to really read things so they have used that to their advantage.

The food industry has become a multimillion dollar industry with branches of it even receiving additional revenue from pesticide and pharmaceutical companies. There are several tactics used to thrill us with our purchases that do more harm than good. The key to all of this is to learn as much as possible so that you can be your own health advocate and make the best possible choices without depending on a store, company or manufacturer to look after your best interest. As women with SuperPowers I want to keep this as simple as possible, since time is of the essence!

Interpreting a Food Label – Food labels are designed to give us healthful information so that we can easily see if the nutrient quantities meet our needs and health. Now here's the reality; food labels can be so easily altered and misread simply by playing with portion sizes and recognizing that anything that is less than 10% of the ingredients doesn't even have to be listed on the label ... hmmm. My goal is to push you to eat as many foods as possible that don't even come with a food label, that come to you in their natural, unaltered state! But for those times when you have no choice or it's a staple pantry item, I really need you to understand how it all works.

Food Label Masquerade

What the food label says and how your body metabolizes it are two totally different things. Something with zero fat grams can still be stored as fat, so don't get fooled! More than likely, most foods with a food label will make you fat if you overindulge.

The %'s used make you feel like you are doing such a great thing with the nutrients in the package, just remember that they use a 2000 calorie plan to create those %'s and 2000 calories of food is A LOT more than some would eat!

Nutrition Facts

Serving Size 1.25 Cup (286g)
Servings Per Container 5

Amount Per Serving	
Calories 310	Calories from Fat 110
	%Daily Value*
Total Fat 12g	**18%**
Saturated Fat 4g	**20%**
Trans Fat 0g	
Polyunsaturated Fat 1g	
Monounsaturated Fat 5g	
Cholesterol 20mg	**7%**
Sodium 290mg	**12%**
Potassium 780mg	**22%**
Total Carbohydrate 36g	**12%**
Dietary Fiber 12g	**48%**
Sugars 6g	
Protein 17g	

Vitamin A 20%	Vitamin C 80%
Calcium 20%	Iron 20%
Vitamin E 8%	Vitamin K 110%
Thiamin 25%	Riboflavin 20%

Calories per serving – What you consider a serving and what the manufacturer considers a serving are two different things. Be sure to understand what the serving size looks like compared to your serving size. Many times they opt for a smaller serving size to highlight the "reduced calories" and so that they don't have to list certain ingredients in the ingredient list.

The DV% represents the % of the total recommended allowance for a specific nutrient, but we all require different amounts so the recommended amount may or may not meet your specific needs.

As for the ingredients list; ingredients are listed in descending order of weight (from most to least). Note that anything below 10% of the total ingredients does not need to be listed on the ingredient list. Manufacturers can hide many unhealthy items under the premise of "Natural Flavors"; this could mean anything from MSG to an array of preservatives. Also, as long at 30% of the ingredients are organic, they can sell the product as "organic". With this said, all ingredients would need to say "organic" and those that don't ... aren't. The best rule to follow when you're checking out a label is if you cannot pronounce it and have no idea what it is, **DON'T EAT IT!**

INGREDIENTS

FILTERED WATER, WHEAT, ORGANIC MALTODEXTRIN, ORGANIC EVAPORATED CANE SUGAR, NATURAL FLAVORS, DIPOTASSIUM PHOSPHATE, SALT, MAGNESIUM CITRATE, CALCIUM LACTATE, BLACKBERRIES.

MAY CONTAIN WHEAT AND NUTS

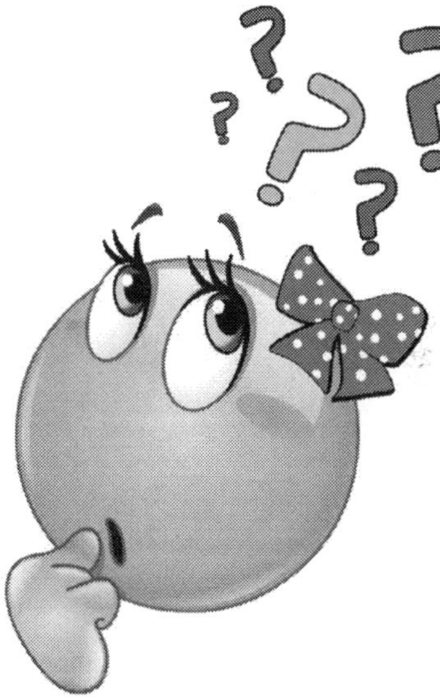

Manufactured and processed foods bring with them more challenges than benefits. Manufacturers have mastered the art of deception in both their packaging and ingredient terminology, making it even more important to understand ingredients, recognize how they affect your health, and not get taken in by the pretty packaging!

Packaging Claims: Packaged and processed foods are filled with a variety of claims and marketing "words" to make you feel like you are making the BEST PURCHASE EVER! Many of these nutritional claims are false. For example, "light" vegetable oil is merely light in color, and "light" cheesecake light in texture. With new labeling, any term used to describe a particular food's nutrient content will have a universal meaning. Unfortunately, the food label can contain just a few ingredients that fit the claim and still highlight it on the packaging. Such words as "organic", "non-GMO", "natural", "free", "low," "light or lite," "immune support", "less," and "high" may or may not be listed correctly.

Not to mention the pretty colors and pictures to make you feel that the package is natural and organic even if it isn't. Imagine this; you go to the store wanting to buy a healthier pancake mix. You look at all the packages on the shelf and one is in a brown bag with a recycled paper label that looks even homemade. Wow, that must be it, look how natural and fresh it makes you feel. The packaging alone just oozes "ORGANIC"—not! This particular package is filled with preservatives, high fructose corn syrup, and a whole host of unmentionables, so don't get duped!

Now, with all this said, how valuable is it to buy organics? Let's start with the icky stuff FIRST... GMO

Genetically Modified Foods – (GMO or engineered foods) – Although this is a fairly new phenomenon, the pesticide industry has gone crazy with all the things that can be engineered. As of today, while I write this book, the industry promotes genetically modified seeds from such crops as sugar beets, corn, soy, and wheat, but I'm sure they are working on others. They have engineered these seeds to withstand high levels of pesticides without killing the crop or they have modified the seed to carry its own internal pesticide so that when a bug tries to eat the plant, the bug dies. The FDA does not require vendors to list ingredients that have been engineered, although some vendors are proud to list that there is "No GMO" in their products. Are these safe choices or not? Research is limited and filled with mixed reviews, the research that does promote GMO typically originates from the pesticide companies or the conventional farmers that use them, so just look at it this way, would you eat an apple that I just sprayed with bug spray? I don't know about you, but with diseases spreading at such a high level, I want to put as few questionable chemicals into my system as possible.

Organics don't look as expensive now, do they?

Organics – This has been the catchphrase for some time now, it basically means that no pesticides were used to grow these foods and that no chemicals were added to the food during processing. The research is limited but there is evidence that organics are farmed in such a manner that the soils are richer in nutrients and provide a higher level of nutrition per bite than their conventional counterparts. On the flip side, many argue that organic farms still receive residue from both GMO and pesticides, but, as I have seen, most farms take the utmost care to assure the quality of their grains or produce. These farmers are proud of their products and proud of their reputation. Either way, the levels of any possible chemical will be much less on an organic farm than a conventional one, don't you think?

Organic vs. Conventional – So what do you do now? Which do you choose? No matter how you look at it conventional fruits and vegetables are sprayed down with a mixed cocktail of chemicals that have been deemed safe by the FDA. The biggest challenge is that the studies used to label these chemicals as safe were performed on an average 150 lb. adult male, so that definitely does not prove they are safe for all of us. I'm sorry but that's not enough proof for me to ingest a chemical cocktail!

Now, not all things are sprayed and some things don't soak it in as much as others, you can get pretty savvy at choosing just the right organics and just the right conventional produce to meet your needs and your pocket book. The pesticides penetrate the produce through the outer layer, so those with thicker skins (i.e. oranges, bananas) may contain lower levels than those with thin or no skins (i.e. strawberries, raspberries). Then there are things like onions that don't usually get sprayed at all. The Environmental Working Group has a wonderful list and app to let you know which to choose from (look for their site in my resources page). Look for the Dirty Dozen and the Clean Fifteen. On that same note there are several co-ops all over the world that sell organics at a "per share" rate and can save you as much as 50% on your organics bill. I love my co-op and it forces me to try some things I would never have delved into before.

Prioritize your staple foods! –
Pesticides add up easily, so keep them ORGANIC.

The easiest way to be sure you are skipping the bad stuff and only buying the good is to know the codes. Here you have them in a nutshell:

Produce Codes Demystified

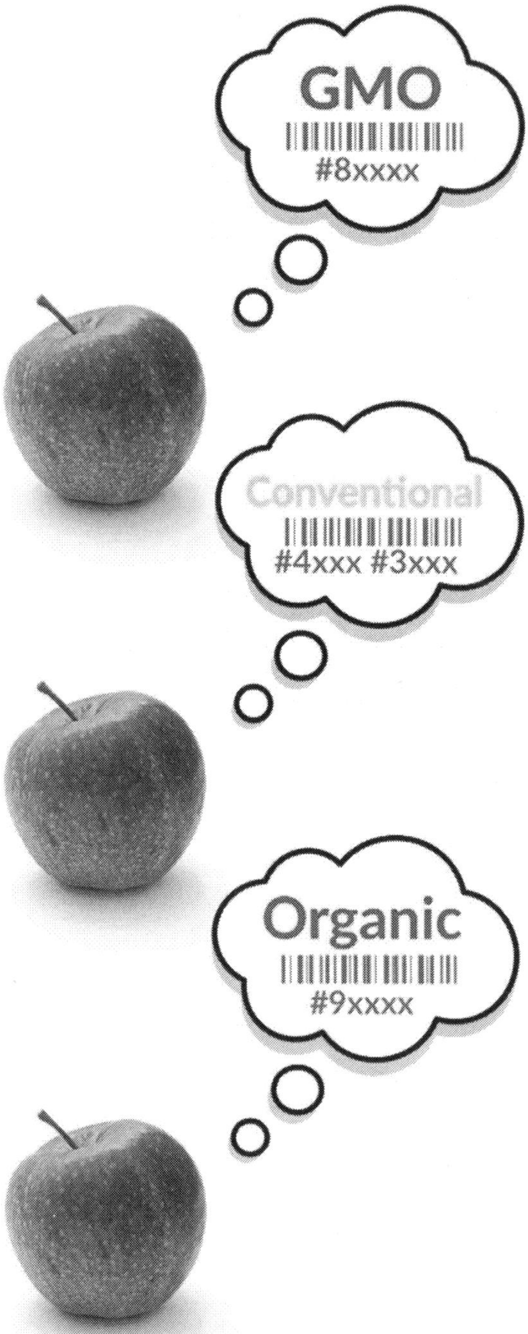

8

Genetically Modified

Avoid these!

3 & 4

Grown with chemicals

Just ok for certain fruits & vegetables

9

Grown without chemicals

Gold Standard

Fortified – Sounds fancy and it sounds like you are just getting this "Mecca" of nutrition with each and every bite. Well, here is how they lay it out, as defined by the World Health Organization (WHO) and the Food and Agricultural Organization of the United Nations (these sound very official, so they must be important). Fortification refers to "the practice of deliberately increasing the content of an essential micronutrient, i.e. vitamins and minerals (including trace elements) in a food irrespective of whether the nutrients were originally in the food before processing or not, so as to improve the nutritional quality of the food supply and to provide a public health benefit with minimal risk to health," whereas enrichment is defined as "synonymous with fortification and refers to the addition of micronutrients to a food which were lost during processing." 80+ years ago, fortification of foods was started to enrich the nutrient content of foods in countries where malnutrition was prevalent.

OK so what does all of this jargon mean? This initially started with foods sent over to impoverished nations as a means of enhancing their nutrients in a "processed food" delivery system. Since they were vitamin deficient from the start, their bodies reveled in the flood of nutrients they were receiving. Today, no matter how badly we eat, we still receive enough nutrients for survival. With this said, "fortified" foods can create a lot of hype and make us feel like we are getting a huge nutritional jolt but with our bodies not starving for nutrition these simply provide us with calories and little to no benefit. Remember these nutrients are synthetically derived nutrients with no enzymes to help out, so our bodies would much rather take nutrients from high quality foods than these "fortified" wannabes!

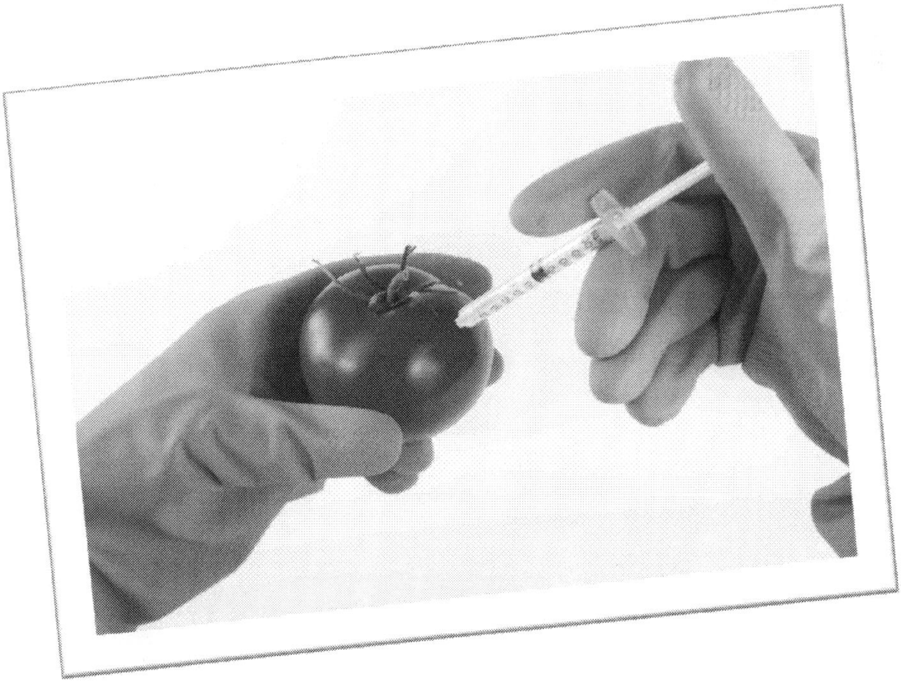

Superfoods –This relatively new term refers to foods that give you large amounts of nutrition per bite or have a high nutritional density. Eat Right America rates the Superfoods by an ERNI Score; Whole Foods Market uses an ANDI Score—either way this helps us identify which fruits or vegetables to choose from for a higher nutritional punch.

Here are my top ten favorites:

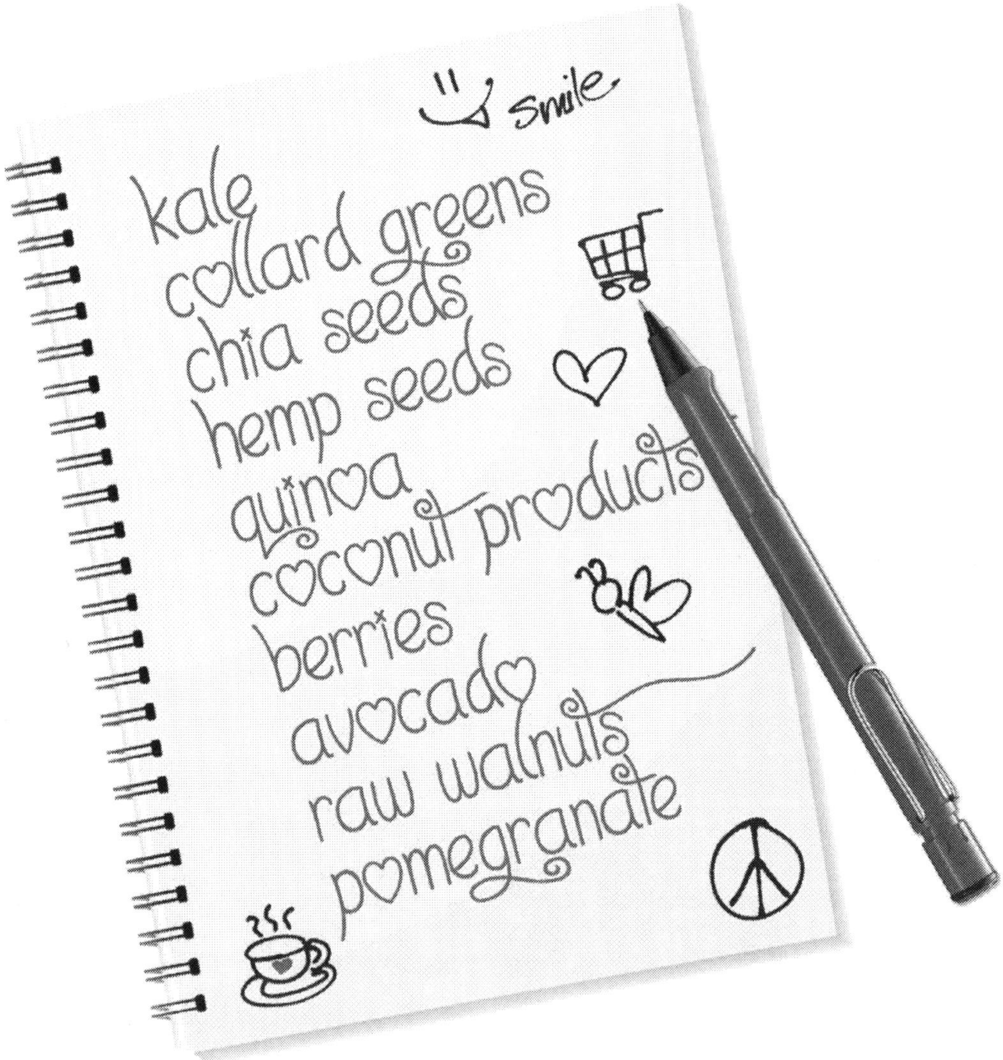

Maximum nutrition in every bite!

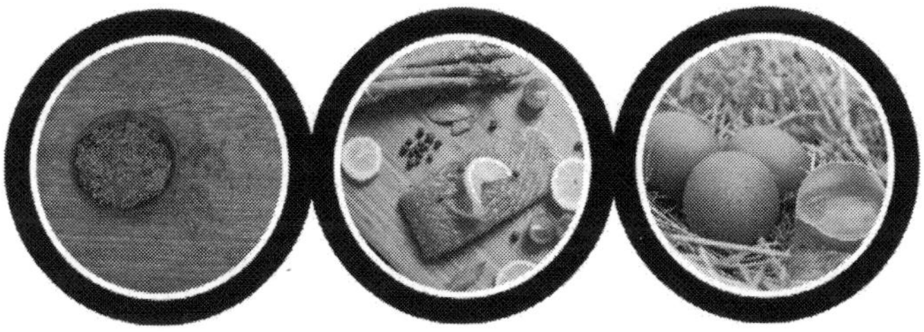

ESSENTIAL FATTY ACIDS

Essential Fatty Acids (EFAs) – High octane for the brain! For our kids this means that their growing brains will receive all the nourishment needed, and for us SuperWomen, this means our brains will be clear, strong, and crystal clear for years to come. So what are the best sources?

Eggs - Not just any ordinary chicken, you want organic, free range, and pasture fed.

Raw Hemp Seeds - This complete protein has little taste and can be easily combined into a salad, smoothie or anything else you can dream of because no one will really know it's there, but your brain will love you for it.

Raw Flaxseeds - These can also be added to just about anything but should be freshly ground before eating.

Salmon or Sardines - Here are the "crown jewels", our bodies assimilate these the best, our challenge is finding sources that are not farmed and are caught swimming wild instead.

Raw Nuts, especially Walnuts - Raw nut butters or freshly chopped raw nuts can be added to just about anything, and don't forget a handful of trail mix, that's a good option as well!

Avocados - This poor fruit has had a bad rap of being fatty. No limits; just enjoy and reap all of the nutritional benefits it provides you with. This guy is so great that you can even use the leftovers for a hair mask or facial!

SUPPLEMENTS

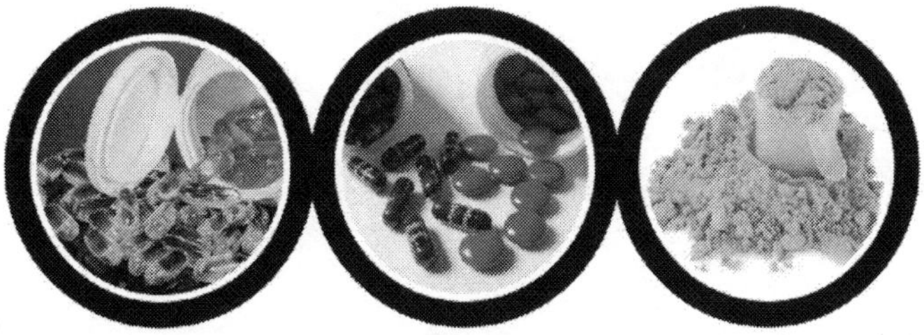

Supplements - They are just that—they supplement your body to provide you with the missing nutrients that, for whatever reason, you simply are not absorbing from your foods. Ideally you should receive everything from your foods; there is that small chance, through added stress or disease that you will be lacking in something. These are the times when you can supplement, but you're better off finding a practitioner to help you choose just the right thing at the right amount, rather than self-medicating.

Supplements can be easily combined incorrectly with other supplements or medications; this is why food is so awesome, we don't have to worry about these kinds of bad combinations. A great practitioner can check out your blood, stool, and urine and see exactly what you need.

There are tons of supplements out there that will promise you the moon! Drop fat instantly, rev up your gears in a minute, and perform feats never seen by the human eye, HA! Girl, it's only a dream, you'll show the world so much more if you just make a few changes to your day and your food plan, just you wait and see.

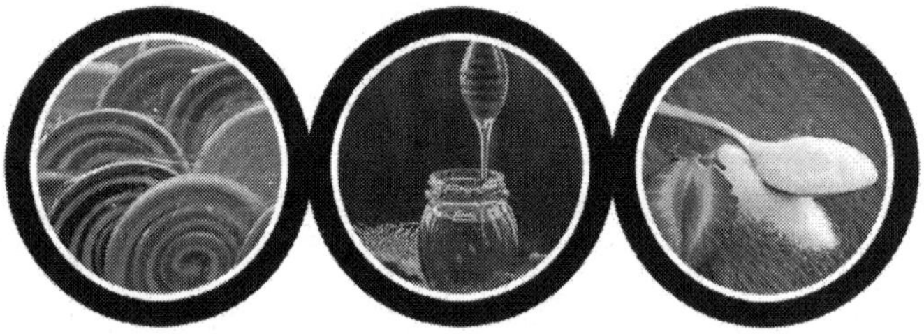

SUGAR

SUGAR, SUGAR, AND MORE SUGAR! – This refers to everything from sugar to stevia, agave, and more, but it is important to recognize that many other things metabolize as a sugar and when too much "sugar" is being processed it is then stored as FAT, slows you down, and hampers clear and powerful thinking. The average consumer consumes 22 teaspoons of sugar per day; the body can safely handle 6 teaspoons of sugar per day. So, with this said, let's talk about all those nasty sweeteners and figure out who is truly our friend:

Hidden terms referring to sugar: There are over 100 names for sugar that are used by manufacturers to hide the fact that they are adding a ton of sugar to your foods. They use such names as malt barley, molasses, brown rice syrup, cane juice, carob syrup, dextran, diastatic malt, and many more to make you believe these are natural ingredients or preservatives. The following are the most common types of sugar and their effects on our health:

Table Sugar (sucrose) – Typically manufactured from sugar beets (which is on our top 5 list of GMO foods). Table sugar is a combination of fructose and glucose (glucose being what we use for energy) and although it provides less fructose than high fructose corn syrup it can break down easier but still with a variety of health concerns. There is no nutritional benefit to table sugar.

Corn Syrup and High Fructose Corn Syrup (HFCS) – These sweeteners are addictive, inexpensive to make, and metabolize as a fructose, which causes stress to the liver. Fructose

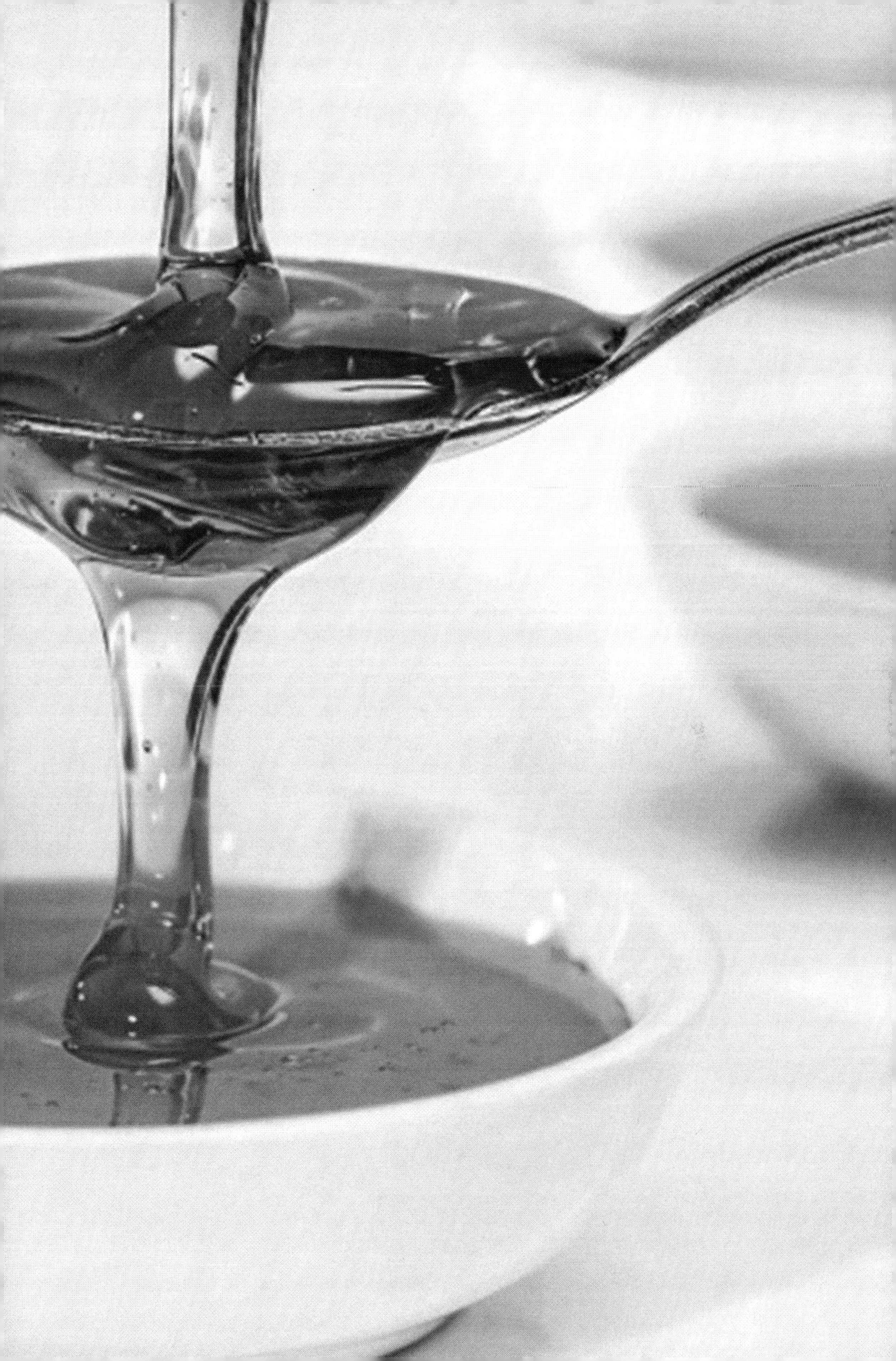

is turned into free fatty acids (FFAs), VLDL (the damaging form of cholesterol), and triglycerides, which get stored as fat and trigger high cholesterol. Additionally, these sweeteners have been linked to high cholesterol, heart disease, diabetes, and obesity. So think twice before driving through and grabbing a soda!

Agave – This is a highly processed sap from a cactus that is *almost all fructose*. Your blood sugar will spike just as it would if you were consuming regular sugar or HFCS. Agave's rise in popularity is due to a great marketing campaign, but any health benefits present in the original agave plant are all processed out.

These are the two best choices when it comes to health, calories, and any nutritional benefits.

Stevia – This is a tea leaf! And when steeped as a tea, it produces a naturally sweet liquid that can be used as a sweetener for just about anything. The challenge arises when it has been over processed and no longer looks like a "tea". With this said, liquid stevia is your best choice, it should have no chemical additives, it naturally has no calories, and little if any side effects.

Honey - This blend of sugar, trace enzymes, minerals, vitamins, and amino acids is quite unlike any other sweetener and brings along an entire list of healthful benefits. Honey still breaks down as fructose but its combination of enzymes, healing and antibacterial properties makes it a much better choice.

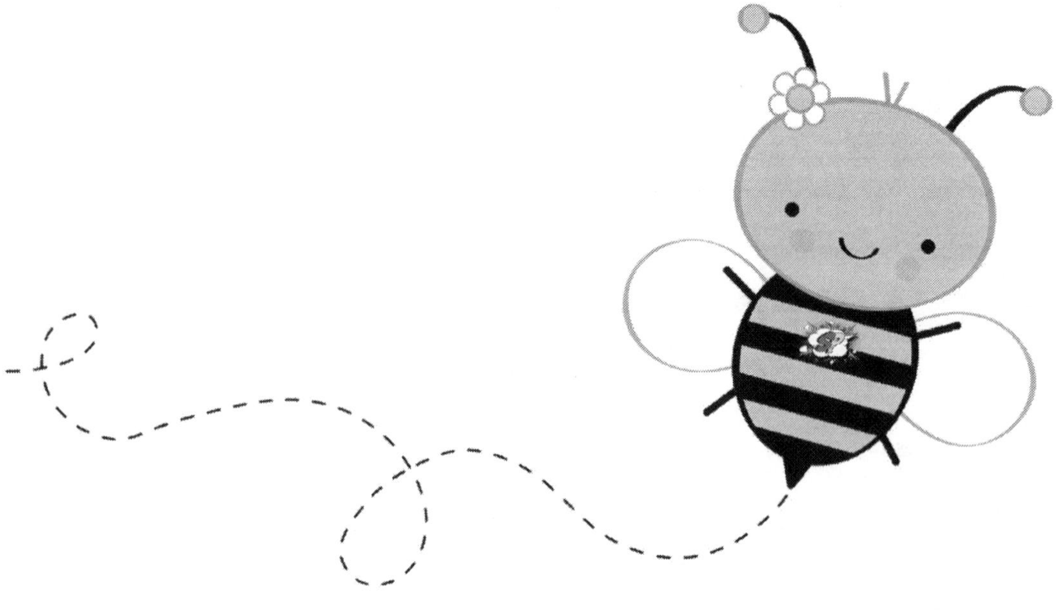

A few more things to keep in mind about SUGAR:

Did you know your immune system can be placed on SNOOZE? With only 8 teaspoons of traditional table sugar, corn syrup, high fructose corn syrup or the like, your immune system can be suppressed up to 40% for 30 minutes all the way to 5 hours. So ... better think twice before indulging with that soda or candy bar or anything else that satisfies your sweet tooth. Remember: Sugar, flour, dairy, and alcohol ALL metabolize as sugar and as a woman with SuperPowers you need to keep your immunity strong, powerful, and invincible!

How fast does the sugar get into your system? The glycemic index is a measure of how quickly a food will increase blood sugar. Simple sugars, such as high fructose corn syrup, quickly flood the blood with fructose and glucose. This puts stress on the body, which attempts to bring blood sugar back to equilibrium. The lower the glycemic index the slower the blood sugar will rise. These foods would need additional protein, fiber, and/or fat in order to slow down the digestive process. With a high glycemic index, foods that are not immediately used for energy are easily stored as fat. A good example of this is a banana, if you eat the banana and work out, chase your kids or go on an errand rampage, the sugar will be used for what you just did and the nutrients absorbed in the body. Now, if you eat a banana, a cookie, and a bowl of pasta and just sit back for the day watching soaps, reading magazines and truly breaking your SuperWoman code of ethics, there is too much sugar in the system and the body will store much of the unused content as fat (and you wonder why we have a code of ethics, ha!).

The Many Faces of SUGAR & Sweeteners

Acesulfame-K ~ AGAVE ~ Aspartame ~ Barley Malt ~ Beet sugar ~ Blackstrap molasses ~ Brown sugar ~ Cane sugar ~ Cane juice crystals ~ CARAMEL ~ Carob syrup ~Castor sugar ~ Coconut Sugar ~ Corn sweeteners ~ Corn Syrup ~ Confectioner's sugar ~ Crystalline fructose ~ Cyclamates ~ Date sugar ~ Demerara sugar ~ Dextrin ~ Dextros ~ Diastatic malt ~ Diatase ~ D-mannose ~ Evaporated cane juice ~ Fructose ~ Fruit juice concentrate ~ Galactose ~ Glucose ~ High-fructose corn syrup (HFCS) ~ Honey ~ Invert sugar ~ Lactose ~ Malt syrup ~ Maltodextrin ~ Maltose ~ Maple syrup ~ Molasses ~ Neotame ~ Raw sugar ~ Rice syrup ~Saccharin ~ Splenda ~ SUCRALOSE ~ SUCROSE ~ Syrup ~ Table sugar ~ Treacle ~ Turbinado sugar

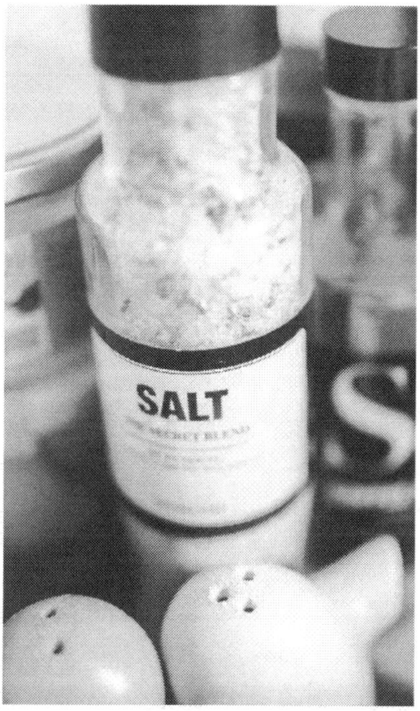

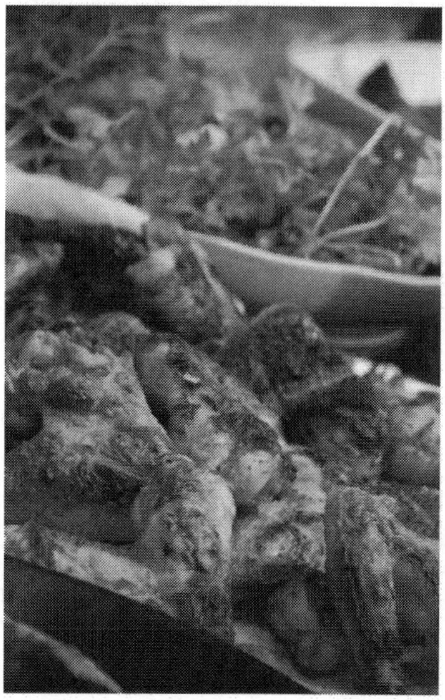

Salt is not a terrible thing. It can actually help you stabilize your energy and calm down your system in times of stress and chaos. The challenges have been the numerous choices that we are surrounded with. Traditional table salt provides the body with no nutritional value and actually strips us of needed nutrients just so the body can metabolize it. Choose salts like Celtic sea salt or Himalayan salt; these taste the same as table salt but are packed with naturally occurring enzymes, minerals and vitamins to keep the body in optimal condition.

Chicken and Meat – Do you buy hormone free, natural or organic or do you choose the best deal in the store?

FYI – If you choose to do neither, your meat or chicken is probably packed with growth hormone and/or antibiotics and they are fed grains that include fillers and genetically modified ingredients. If this hasn't convinced you to go organic yet, would this sound appealing? Arsenic, antibiotics, growth hormones, pesticides, and whatever else is available to enhance the density and appearance of ... conventional chicken. I realize cost may be a factor, but if you educate yourself enough and understand the quality of various food items, you'll be able to choose organic for the things that could most affect the health of you and your family and choose conventional for anything else or for those house guests you really don't care about.

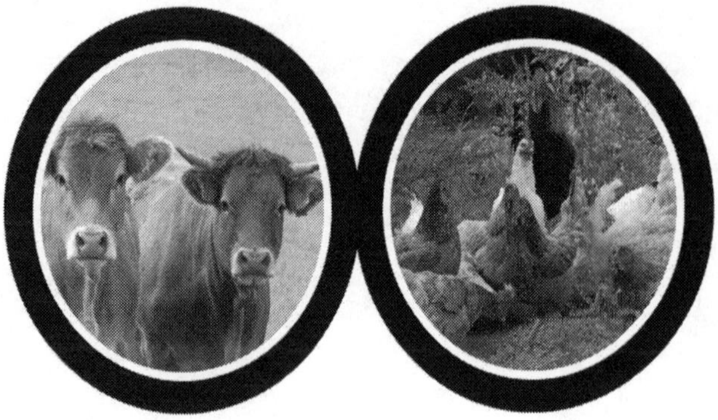

SUPERPOWER STRONG

- Organic grass fed/grass finished butter, dairy products, beef, and ghee
- Organic pasture fed/free range poultry and eggs
- Organic grass fed beef
- Organic free range poultry and eggs
- Non organic 100% grass fed/grass finished beef
- Non organic free ranged poultry and eggs
- Non organic grass fed/grain finished beef
- Conventional poultry and eggs
- Conventional dairy (including cheese, milk, ice cream, yogurt, and creamers)
- Conventional and packaged meats and poultry

ONLY FOR THE WEAK

Organic – This means that no drugs were used on the animals and that all the feed is clean of pesticides or genetically modified crops. The key here is to also recognize if they are vegetarian fed or naturally fed, animals do better eating what they want, how they want it, rather than a prepared meal by some scientific guru.

Free range, organic, grass or pasture fed – This is the "golden ticket" of fine poultry and meat. These are organic, they roam freely in their natural environment, and they eat from their natural food source without any alterations.

Natural – The animals were fed natural grains, which aren't necessarily their food of choice, with no fillers or by-products, but the grains are not organic and they are more than likely genetically modified. Also, unless otherwise specified, they could have been given hormones and/or antibiotics.

Hormone /Antibiotic Free – They used no drugs to "plump" up the meat or produce extra milk. With chickens they used no drugs to "plump" up the chicken or to produce more eggs than natural. Also no antibiotics are used to kill off bacteria, etc. But what they eat is a different story.

SUPERPOWER TIP: Most toxins are stored in the fat cells of meat and chicken, so if organic is not an option … cut that icky stuff OFF!

100% Grass Fed – When it comes to meat, this is your meat of choice. There is one catch, not all grass fed beef is 100% grass fed. Many ranchers finish off their beef with either hay or grains, which will impact the nutritional value of the beef, milk, cheese, and butter. So when choosing your meat and dairy, aim for organic and 100% grass fed/grass finished, this will keep your systems strong and powered!

Wild Game – Sounds intimidating, but it is one of the better bets. These are free roaming animals, no drugs, they eat their natural diet, and they run free. They are mainly sold from specialty ranches across the country (unless your husband or you own a gun and hit the Wild West at times) and are packaged without any additional preservatives or chemicals that you would find in the grocery store.

Fish – Fish provides a wonderful amount of protein and an ideal amount of essential fatty acids, unfortunately Mercury and PCBs put a damper on many of our choices. Mercury's toxicity can take up to a year to remove from the system. According to the U.S. Environmental Protection Agency, a safe level of mercury consumption is 1.51 micrograms per day. The average can of tuna has 52.7 micrograms of mercury per gram. The best situation is to include small amounts of fish in your food plan as opposed to utilizing fish as your main source of protein. The wrong types of fish can bring on some crazy health effects that we SuperWomen just don't have time for, such as impaired neurological development in the fetus, cancer, impairment of the peripheral vision, disturbances in sensations, lack of coordination of movements, Alzheimer's, impairment of speech, hearing, walking and muscle weakness. Shrimp, canned light tuna, salmon, pollock, and catfish contain small amounts of mercury, but larger fish such as shark, swordfish, king mackerel, or tilefish contain the highest levels of mercury and should be avoided. One more thing to keep in mind with fish is that "farm raised" means that they are basically living and breeding in their own "stuff", ideally there is wild farmed, these have moving water but are still fed a manufactured meal. On the other hand, WILD is really the best option and, although we are dealing with polluted waters and other toxins, there are some great benefits to be gained from wild caught fish as long as it is only a small part of your food plan.

Dairy (milk, cheese, yogurt, etc. all the yummy staples that many of my SuperWomen survive on) – As I mentioned in the sugar section of this book, dairy metabolizes or "breaks down" as a sugar. The majority of dairy products in the USA are pasteurized, which means that they have been heated at extremely high temperatures to kill off any so-called "bacteria"; unfortunately, this also kills off some of the amazing nutrients and enzymes that dairy provides. Now, if you're lucky enough to live on a farm then ... have at it, you can't go wrong getting it directly from the cow. Most pasteurized dairy is "fortified" with nutrients by a chemist and provides little if any protein. If chosen as a food source it should be eaten in small portions, 100% grass fed, and raw, more as a treat than a main staple!

Acid vs. Alkaline – You will be hearing more and more about this for years to come. Processed foods, dehydration, and a wide array of others will create acid in our bodies—disease and cancer LOVE ACID. So the key here is to keep a higher alkaline to acid ratio (6.5-7 pH) by eating plenty of fruits and vegetables, drinking lots of water, and choosing foods for the nutrients they can give you. You can easily purchase pH strips from your local pharmacy and check how you're doing with your first morning "pee". It's a great way of making sure that you are staying on the right track for your SuperPower health!

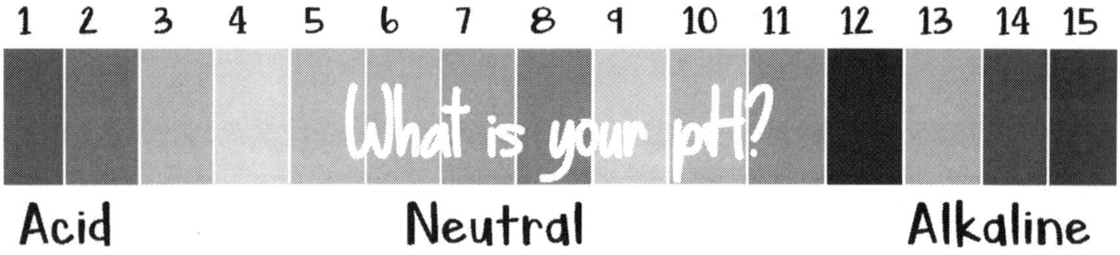

Acid Forming Foods	Alkaline Forming Foods
Meat	Fruit
Fish	Vegetables
Chicken	Lentils
Eggs	Spices
Grains (rice, wheat, corn)	Fresh Herbs & Seasonings
Processed Foods	Raw Nuts and Seeds

Leafy Greens - How many greens have you had today? Yes, greens, green leafy vegetables that are packed with essential nutrients, fiber, and protein. These guys are your friends, they are not here to terrorize you, and actually they are likely to give you a spring in your step and a charge to your battery. If you can't get in that salad, try mixing in some kale or collard greens next time you make a smoothie. It may sound strange, but it's a great way to pack in the nutrients and with the right amount of fruit you won't even know it's there!

Intestinal Health has become a huge business these days; processed foods have disrupted our intestinal flora and have made way for a breeding ground of bad bacteria, bad digestion, unwanted gas, and an array of other icky things. Probiotics is essentially "good bacteria" and it assists the body in combating the bad bacteria and bringing back good health to the digestive tract. A healthy digestive tract will help the body in assimilating all of the wonderful nutrients from our foods and making sure they are available for all of our SuperPower needs. You can supplement your probiotics or you can add fermented foods and beverages such as kimchee, sauerkraut or kombucha to amp up the good guys.

Adrenal Glands – Wakey, wakey; you need to pay attention to this one. As women with SuperPowers we can easily become fatigued, your adrenals can slow down every inkling of progress to your day. Did you know that your adrenal glands are your "energy regulators"? These glands can provide you with unlimited energy throughout the day as long as you take good care of them. The best way to do this is to get adequate rest at night and avoid foods and beverages that provide a "false sense of energy", such as flour, sugar, dairy, alcohol, and caffeine. That's right; your traditional "go to" foods like that bagel may be altering your energy level for your entire day. Since flour, dairy, alcohol, and sugar all metabolize like a sugar they create a type of "energy spike", and the amount of sugar involved will determine how high the spike is. With each spike comes a fall, and some falls are bigger than others. You should have an even amount of energy throughout the day no matter what level of SuperPowers you have; if you find yourself falling asleep at your desk or taking a quick shut eye on top of the washing machine around that 3:00 p.m. hour, your adrenal glands may be sleeping on the job and looking for a bit of TLC from you.

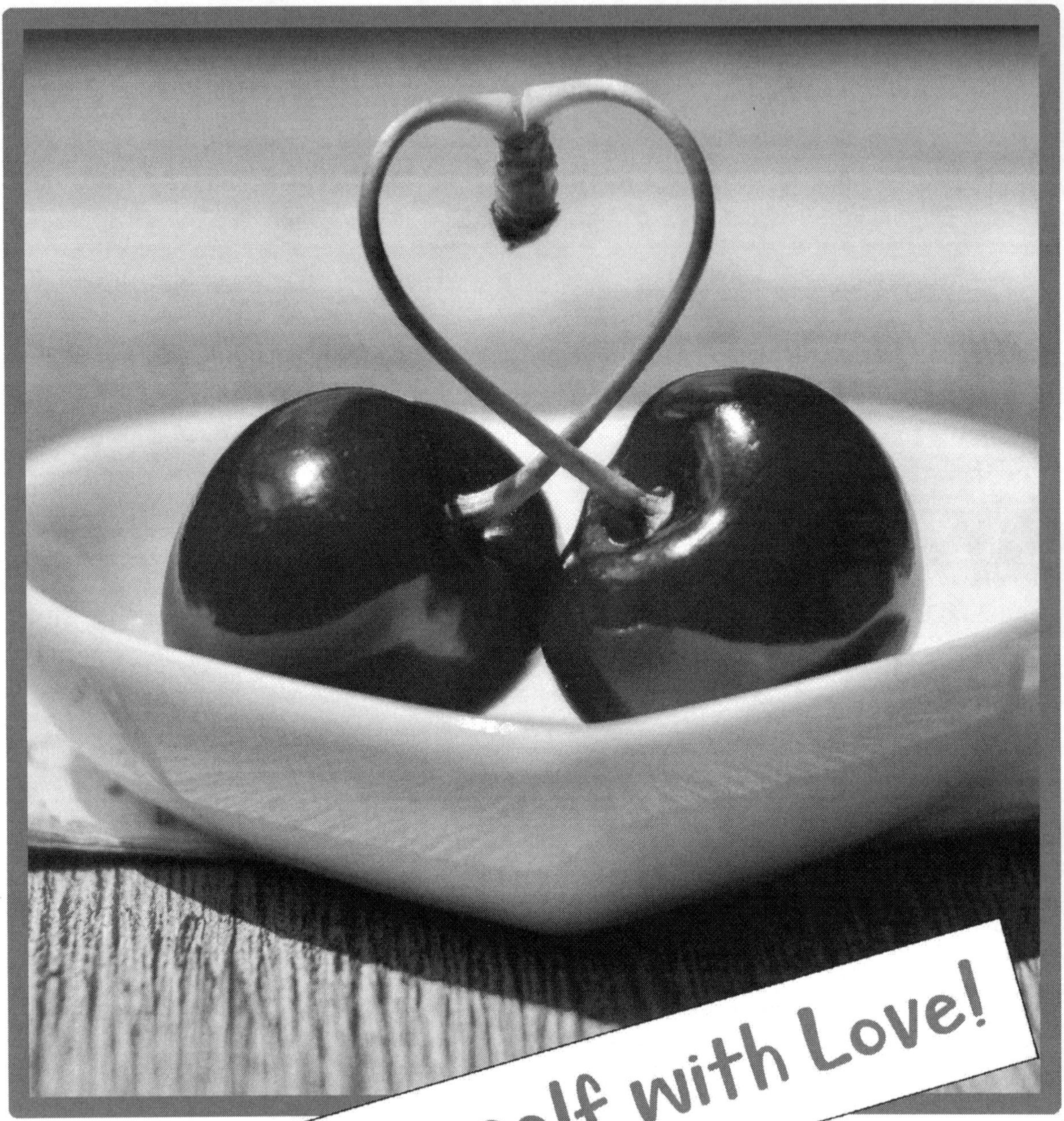

Feed yourself with Love!

"Food is fuel. What you eat today, dictates your health and energy for your entire week, month, and year. Feed yourself with love and nutrition!"

-Adita Lang ♡

p

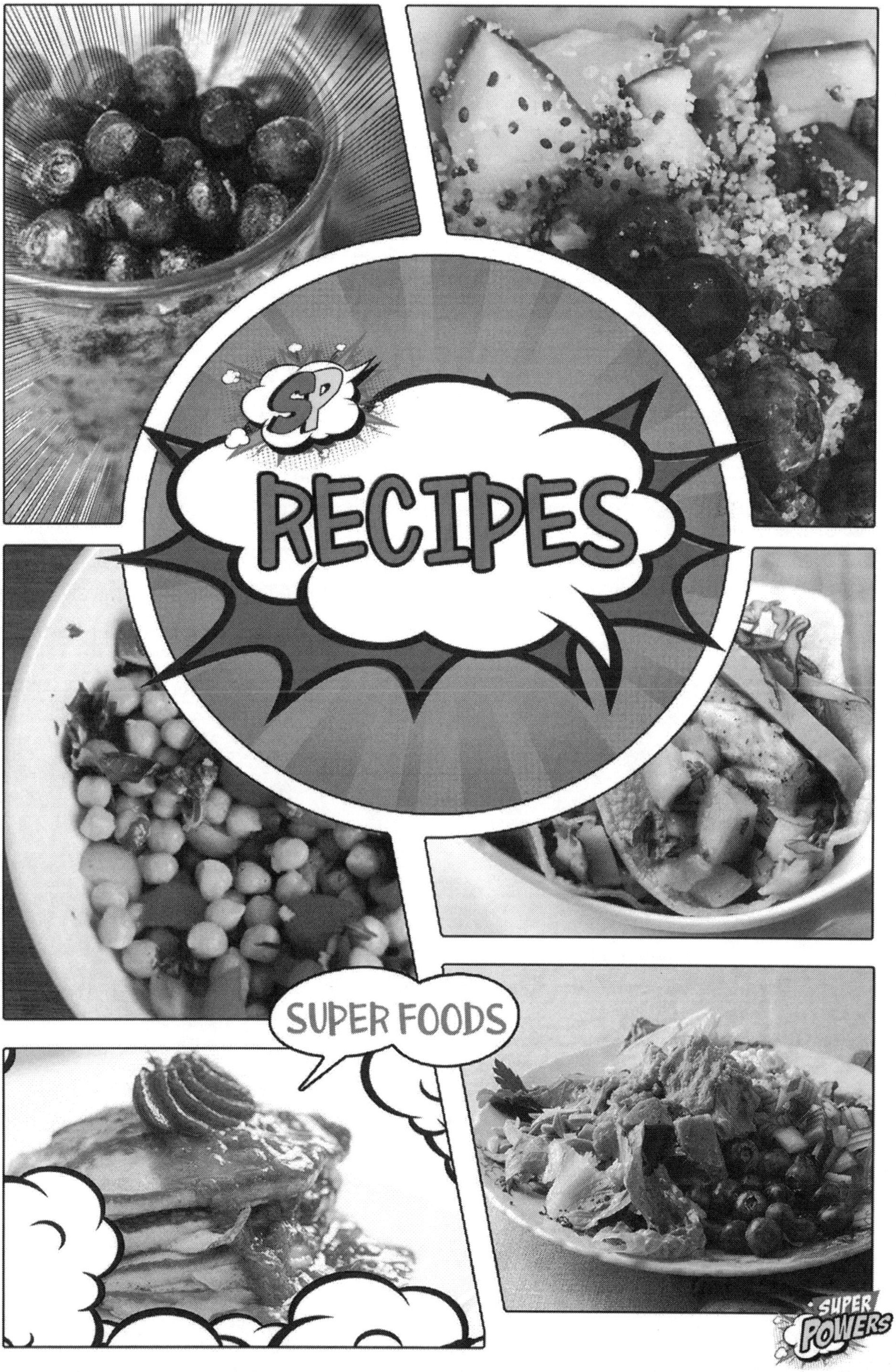
SP
RECIPES
SUPER FOODS
SUPER POWERS

Your Personal Livet® for Taking the World by Storm!

There are no diets here, leave those to the ones who want to torture themselves on an unsuccessful rollercoaster. I am talking about a food plan, and not just any food plan but a Lifetime Food Plan, about eating for whole food nutrition, and about creating the right food plan that you can easily maneuver and use during your perfect day and your most chaotic one! Listen, I realize that you may or may not possess the skills of Betty Crocker® herself or the ultimate Pinterest® mom. Life gets crazy and we just have to go with it, the key is to have the right tools so that we don't get torn down in the process.

As individuals we all metabolize foods differently and due to our individual biochemistry we all have very individual nutritional needs. The one thing that is clear is that the food choices you make can add to your health or add to your weight gain, weight loss, major crankiness, fuzzy brain, and a whole host of additional dumb issues that affect your health and energy. I want to teach you how to create your own perfect Livet®. Now, if you're wondering what that is, let's just compare it to the word "diet", umm, can you see that word "die" in there? We don't like that! Now look at the word "Livet®", so this is a food plan for "living", got it?

Let's get started. There are a few things we are going to set up:

1. You need meals for those times when you are sitting in the car, racing to the office before the boss gets there. We are going to call these your **Emergency Power Meals** or **EPM** for short.
2. **Everyday Food** - You need meals for those days that just seem to flow, the times when you are actually eating with the family and enjoying pleasant conversation.
3. You need snacks for those times when you have run out of fuel and if you don't eat something fast you will buy not one but two dozen freshly baked donuts with sprinkles on top. For ease of classification we will call these your **SuperSnacks.**

4. You need every day snacks to keep your metabolism revved up and your energy on an even keel, **SnackPacks.** A wonderful fast food for our needs is sushi, you can now order it from the deli counter of just about any supermarket, granted most put sugar in the rice but it still wins over any other fast food alternative. Fish needs to be consumed immediately; veggies can last in the car for a while.
5. Beverages, this gets a bit crazy but here is the brunt of it. We need to keep you hydrated, you might need a drink or two to give you an extra leap in your step (and ladies, I am not talking alcohol here, yet it may be appropriate at time, I'm talking for hydration!) and you may need a drink or two to end your day without killing someone, so we will have a section for this too. Let's call these your **Liquid Elixirs.**

Emergency Power Meals (EMP for short)	**Every Day Foods**	**SuperSnacks**	**SnackPacks**	**Liquid Elixirs**
Hard Boiled Eggs	Quinoa with mixed berries and a drizzle of honey	Raw Food Bar	Trail Mix	Coconut Water
Smoothie with Protein	Salad with mixed vegetables, chopped nuts, and chicken or fish	Dates with Almond Butter	Vegetable Sushi Roll (if you can eat it fresh you can have the fish, if not veggies last well in the car)	Herbal Tea or Herbal Chia Late with Almond or Hemp Milk
Protein Pancakes	Quinoa with chopped vegetables and olive oil	Salad in a Jar	Fresh Berries and Raw Nuts	Kombucha
Cut Apple with Almond Butter	Beans and rice with chopped greens and tomatoes	Oatmeal in a Jar	Hummus and Cut veggies	Water with Lemon
Oatmeal in a Jar	Grilled chicken, fish or meat with veggies	Raw Almond Butter and Honey Sandwich	Celery Sticks stuffed with Raw Nut Butter and topped with Goji Berries	Fresh Juice – By fresh I mean you are squeezing it now or watching the person squeeze it

Grab and Go Meal Samplers

These are your primary food categories, yours and only yours. These are the categories for a true SuperWoman, one who has to eat in strange places or on the go! As a true SuperWoman, time is of the essence and although our workouts will also be discussed on another page, we need to eat so that our metabolism is going strong and turns us into a calorie-burning machine. This is where GRAZING comes into play, and I don't mean eating grass from the fields like a cow would. By grazing I mean eating several small meals or snacks per day throughout the day. Our metabolism is that thing that burns extra calories doing ordinary tasks, it's kind of like a light switch and the two things that turn it on the best are food and exercise. So from this point on, you really will not have any distinction between a snack and a meal during your normal day-to-day craziness. Now, granted, you will have those days when "time actually stood still" and you will sit down to an amazing meal and for those moments enjoy them, but for the rest of the time, when eating on the toilet is the only peace and quiet you have, let's make great choices to keep you on schedule.

RECIPE KEY

- GF Gluten Free
- V Vegetarian
- DF Dairy Free
- NS No Sugar
- 15 Prep Time

SUPERPOWER TIP: Every good food plan deserves a few sub categories to help you choose the right things for your health and energy needs. Here are my favs to make this journey easier for you.

Choose the Right Beverage

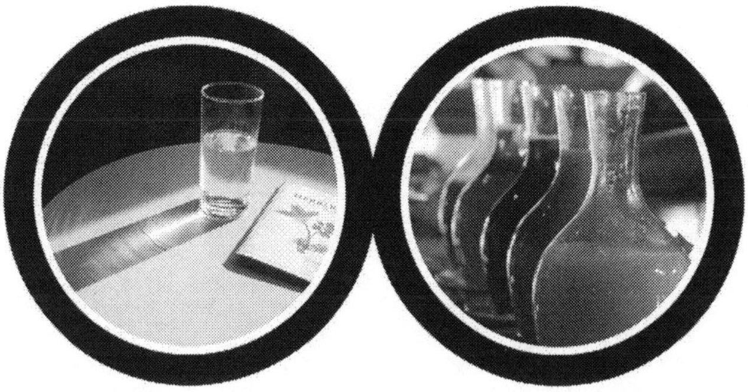

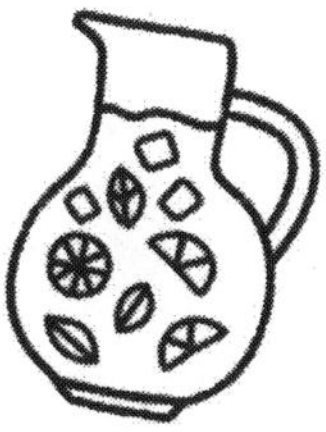

SUPERPOWER STRONG ▲

- Organic raw coconut water
- Organic green tea and coffee
- Filtered water with lemon
- Organic kombucha
- Organic freshly squeezed juice
- Organic raw nut milks
- Tap water or sparkling water with lemon
- Chai latte, coffee, and cappuccinos
- Boxed/pasteurized coconut water
- Pasteurized milk
- Bottled juice
- Soda and diet drinks
- Soy and conventional nut milks
- Sweetened beverages and sport drinks
- Alcohol

▼ ONLY FOR THE WEAK

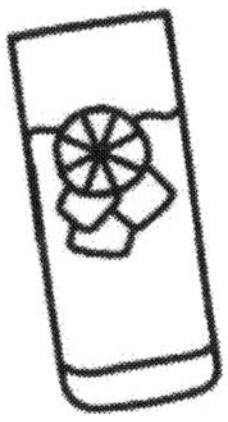

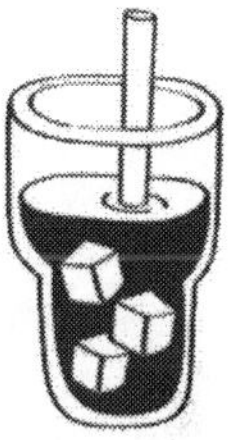

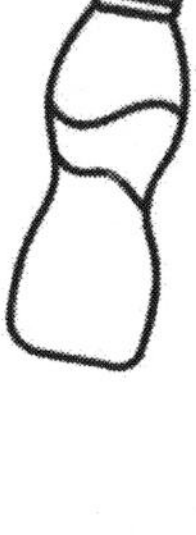

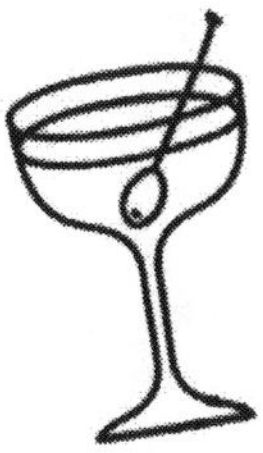

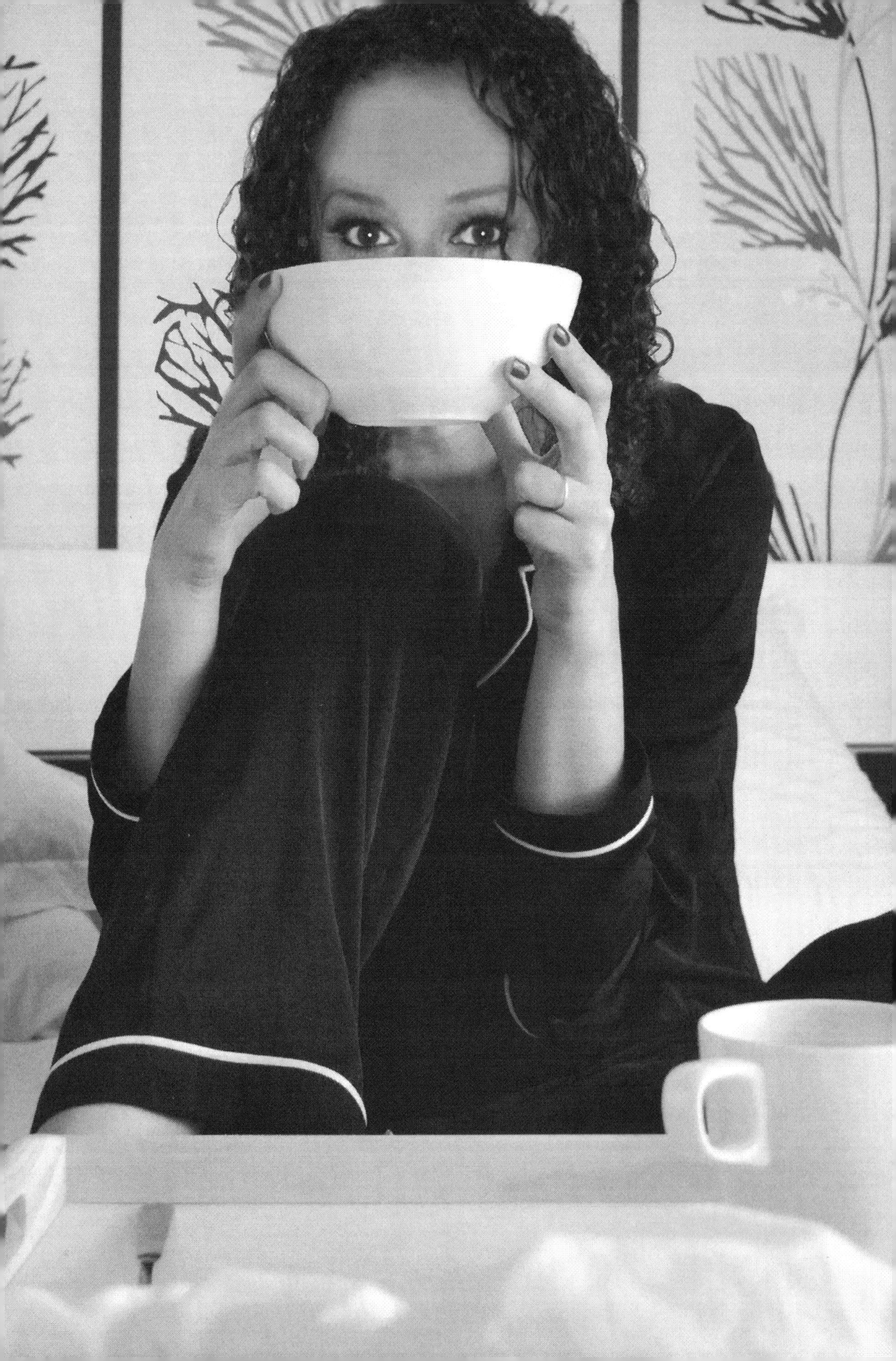

SUPER POWERS

BREAKFAST

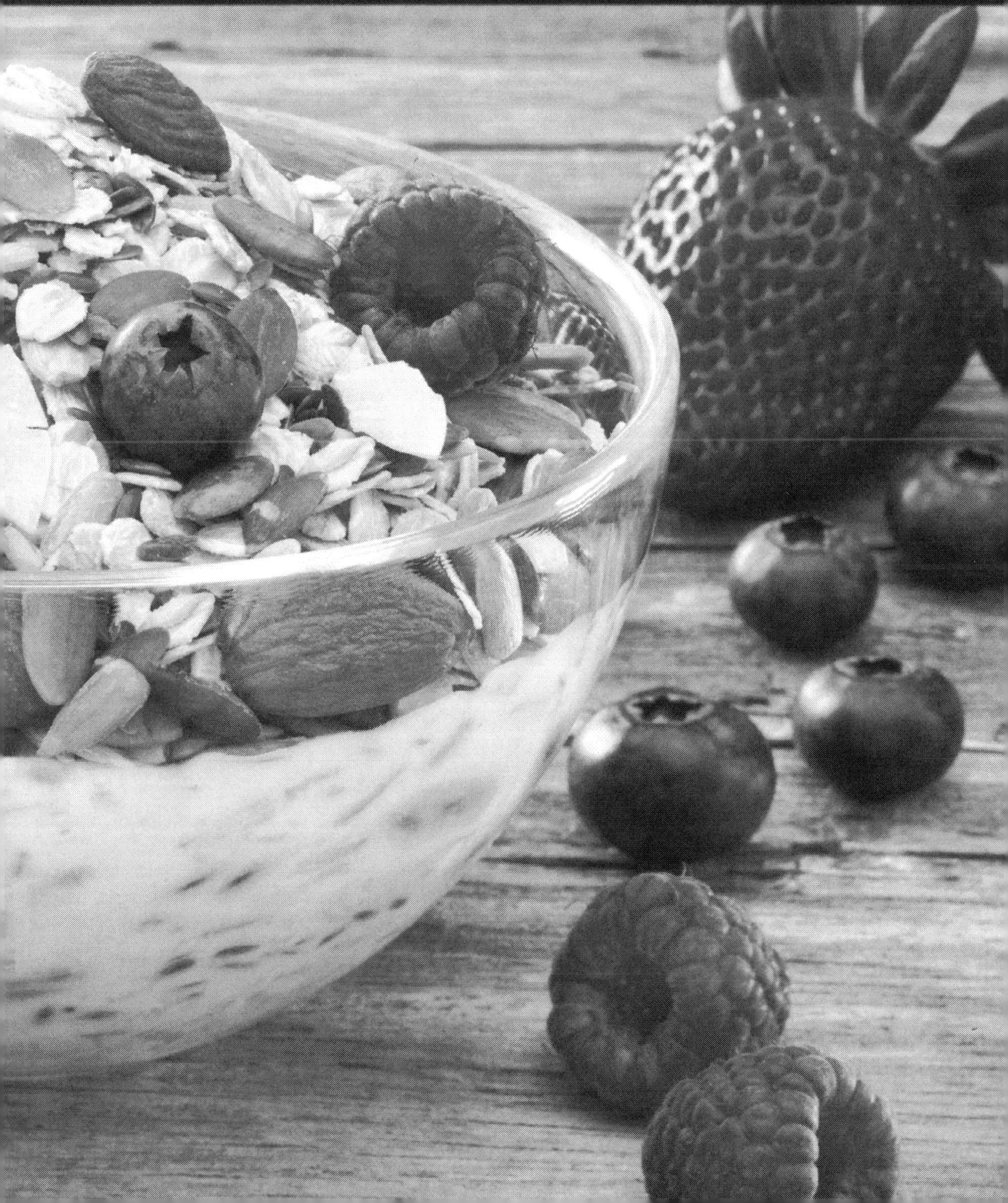

What's for Breakfast?

First thing in the AM: Let's flush out all the toxins that have been sitting in your system all night and get the engines going; start out with two big glasses of water. Now, if your household is like mine, mornings are crazy with 10 different schedules, food requests and just basic organization for everyone's day. Sitting down for breakfast is a true luxury, so, with this said, let's try to start our day with a protein rich treat. Your goal is to have a higher proportion of protein, a little bit of fat, and some quality carbohydrates from fruits, vegetables or grains. Remember, the longer the time until your next meal the more protein and fat this meal should include. This will keep you feeling fuller longer. Some of my favorite "go-to" recipes are:

My Top Picks!

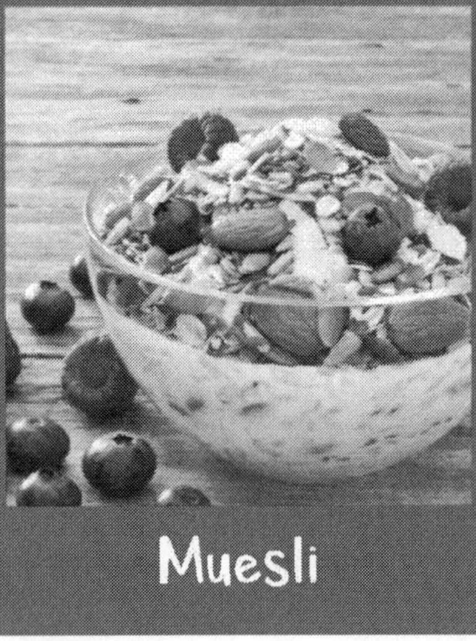

Muesli

DF GF V 15i

Here's a Breakfast that will give you a good amount of quality protein, fats, and carbs, for sustained energy and endurance of your day! Once combined, you can eat it with dairy milk (but remember this is a sugar) or one of the great nut milks that are available.

Ingredients:

Oats
Walnuts
Sliced almonds
Pumpkin Seeds
Sunflower Seeds
Dried mulberries
Goji berries
Coconut Flakes
Cinnamon

Directions:

Mix in a big bowl and serve with milk. Get creative – you can mix just about any dried ingredient (just make sure they don't add any sugar or unidentifiable ingredients), there is rolled barley, rolled rye, raisins, etc. and even combine some fresh ones while you are serving it like berries or chopped apple. Just be sure to have ample protein ingredients, this is where your raw nuts and seeds come in.

SUPERPOWER TIP: Make a big batch and store in an airtight jar for up to a month or set yourself up with a Muesli Bar (airtight jars with each ingredient so that you can create your own mix each and every time).

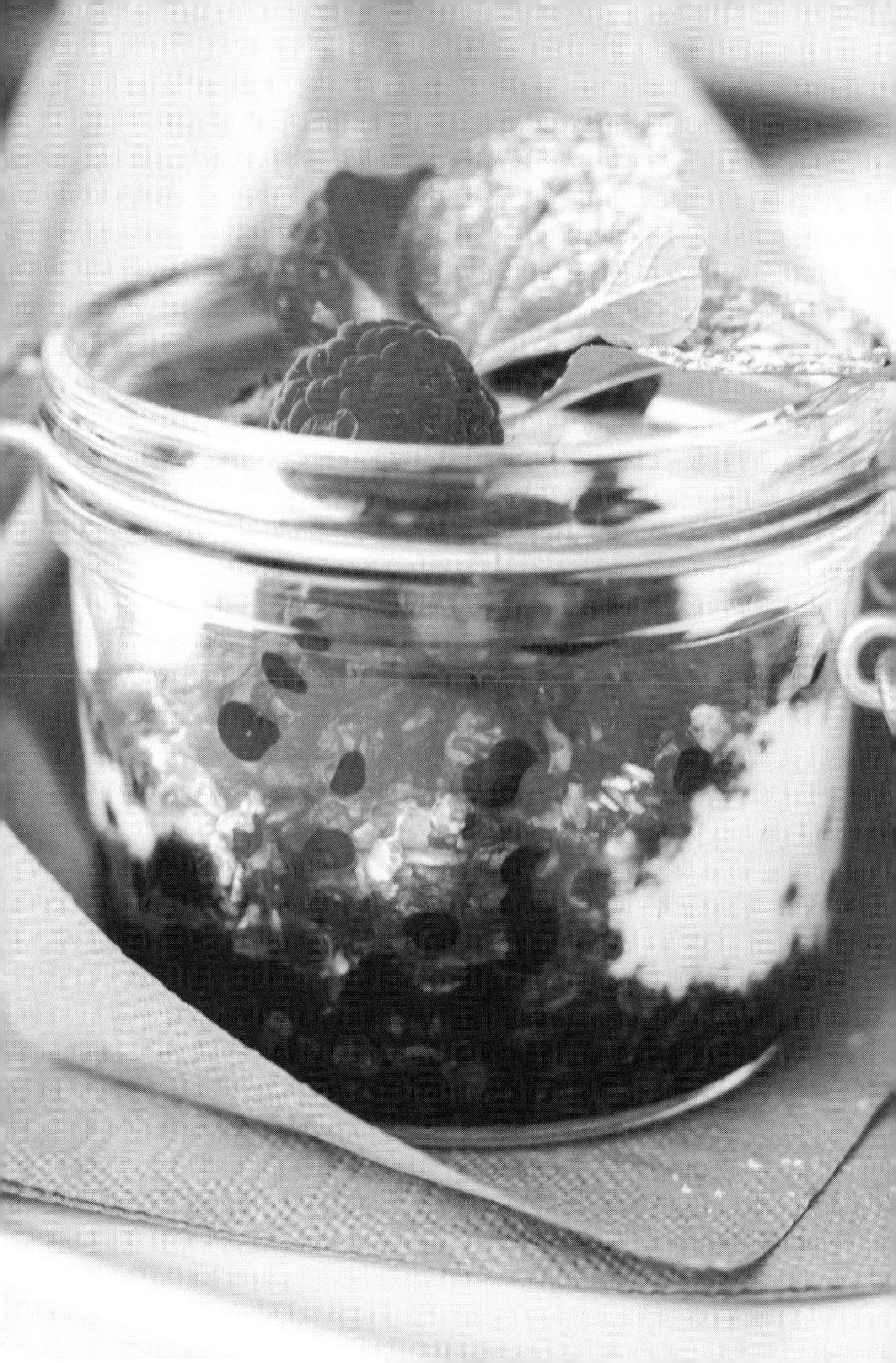

SuperPower Overnight Oats Cheat Sheet

Here's the easiest way of packing in the nutrients into a "fast food", "grab when you need it" type package!

Make your own creation with these guidelines:

1. **Start with Rolled Oats.** Add these in with an equal amount of your liquid of choice. You can use any combination of almond, hemp, or coconut milk; you can even use water but be sure to add in a few more berries for flavor and sweetness if you go the water route. For this rolled oats seem to work best, you can use steel cut oats but you would need to add in more liquid and be prepared to do some extra chewing.

2. **Next Up add in your Flavors.** Here is where you can add in spices like cinnamon and vanilla, even shredded coconut makes it yummy. Also you could add in a scoop of protein powder to give it an extra boost. Pureed dates, honey or stevia and any combination of berries you would enjoy will sweeten it up nicely.

3. **Top it off and Eat up!** For your grand finale add in nut mix (the recipe for this is coming up in the next few pages) or sliced nuts and store in a glass jar or airtight container and let the oats soak for at least three hours, ideally overnight.

SUPERPOWER TIP: If you want to create a few days' worth, then soak only the oats and add in the toppings as your racing out the door. This works great with recycled almond butter jars.

Orange Vanilla Overnight Oats DF GF V

So very yummy!

1. **Start** with your oats but this time, soak them in freshly squeezed orange juice.
2. **Next layer** add in Vanilla as your spice of choice and layer in Coconut Flakes, Nut Mix, and Fruit such as Sliced Mango and Oranges. (You can easily add in protein powder for an extra ounce of fuel!)
3. **Refrigerate**

Maple Almond Butter Overnight Oats DF GF V

1. **Start** with your Oats and Almond Milk
2. **Next layer** comes about 1 tablespoon of Chia Seeds, some Cinnamon, and a dash of Vanilla
3. **Refrigerate**, then when you're about to serve mix one banana with a heaping tablespoon of Raw Almond Butter and add that to the oats. Top it off with a drizzle of maple syrup and a few pecans and you are set.

Coconut Mango Overnight Oats DF GF V

1. **Start** with your Oats and Almond, Hemp or Coconut Milk
2. **Next layer**, a sprinkle of Cinnamon, chopped Mango, a tablespoon of Hemp Seeds, and shredded Coconut. Add in a scoop of protein powder to give it an extra boost, and top that off with sliced Almonds, a drizzle of honey and you are set.
3. **Refrigerate**

SUPERPOWER TIP: I would think by now you are getting the drift of things, we can't let our blood sugar drop and processed carbs don't last long in our system and will exhaust us quicker than you can imagine. I am reiterating it again but I want it ingrained in your head, with everything we do in a day we need tons of naturally occurring nutrients, protein, and a bit of quality fat.

How to cook Quinoa

- ✓ Rinse Quinoa to get rid of bitter taste using a strainer
- ✓ For every 1 cup of quinoa add in 2 cups of water
- ✓ Add a pinch of salt to the top of the water and bring to a boil
- ✓ Cover and reduce heat to low and let stand for 10 minutes
- ✓ Fluff with a fork and serve

Quinoa Morning Eye Opener

Put in a scoop of plain cooked Quinoa into a cereal bowl add in fresh cut fruit and berries and drizzle with a bit of honey

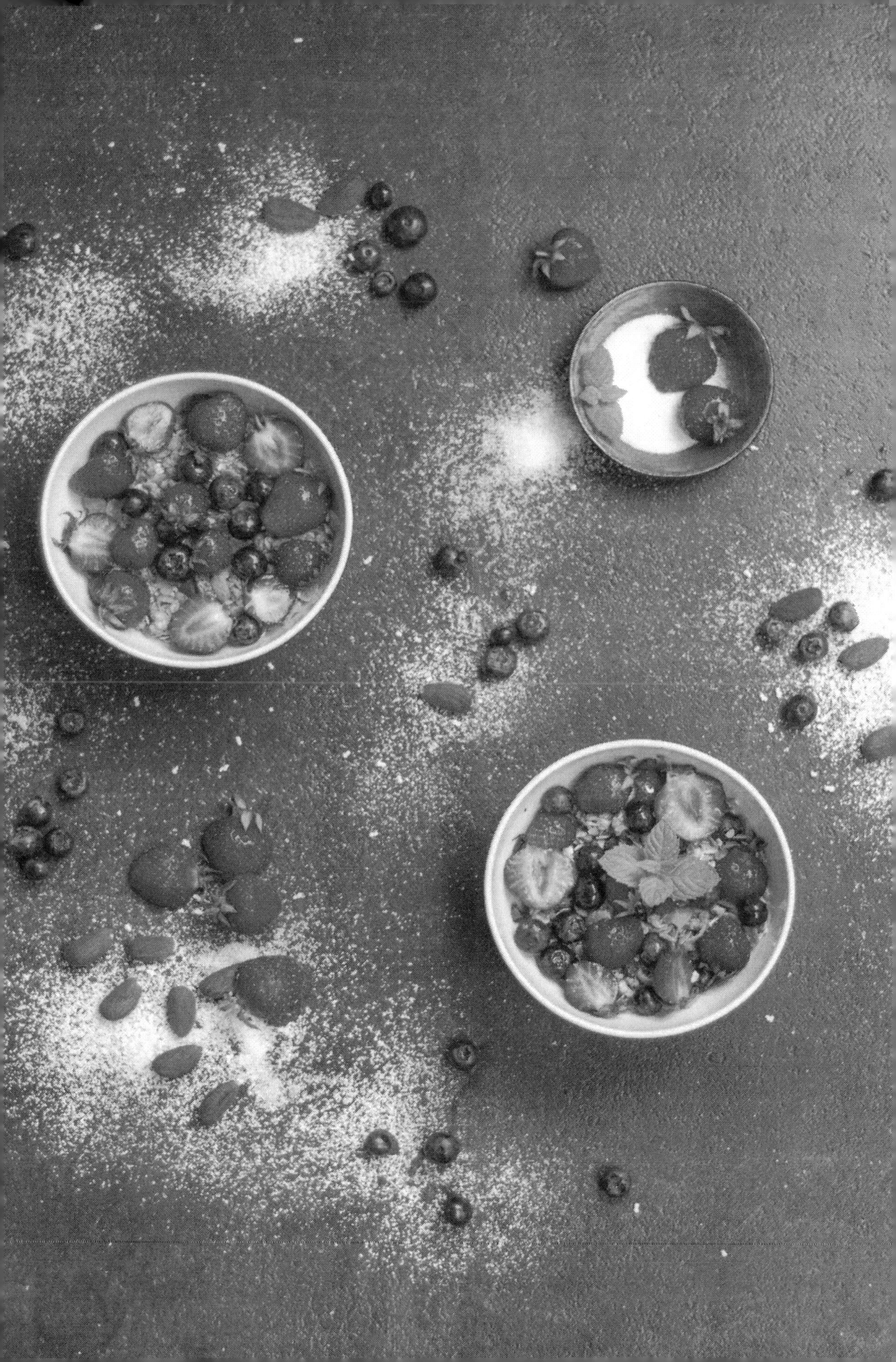

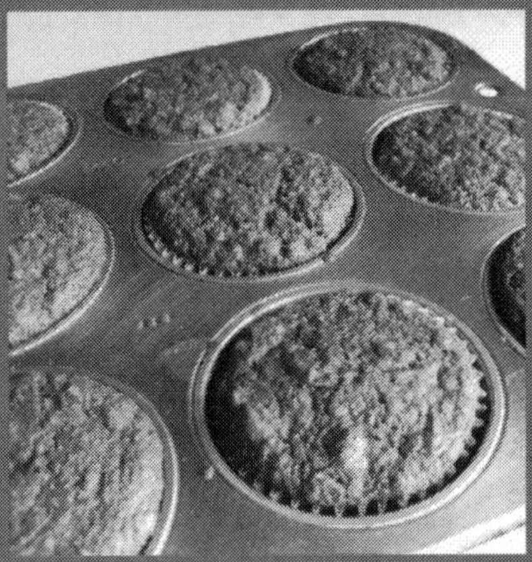

Protein Muffins

Protein Packed Muffins are one of those great inventions that you can hide all sorts of wonderful things in as long as they are sweet!

Ingredients: DF GF V

3 Cups grated fresh Zucchini
1/2 Cup Coconut Oil
11 Medjool Dates (blended with water until smooth)
2 teaspoons Maple Syrup
2 Eggs, (beaten)
2 teaspoons Vanilla
2 teaspoons Baking Soda
Pinch of Celtic Sea Salt
½ Cup Oat Flour and ½ Cup Coconut Flour
2 teaspoons Cinnamon
1/2 teaspoon Nutmeg
1/2 Cup Adita's Nut Mix
1 Cup Mulberries (soaked in water until soft)

Directions:

1. Pre-heat oven to 350 degrees. In a large bowl combine the pureed dates, maple syrup, eggs, and vanilla. Stir in the grated zucchini and the coconut oil. In a separate bowl, mix the flour, baking soda, nutmeg, and cinnamon. Stir everything in together and add in mulberries.

2. Coat Muffin or bread pan with coconut oil and fill the cups up completely with batter. Bake on middle rack until golden brown and poke with a toothpick to make sure the inside is dry. Once cooked, remove from oven and let cool for about five minutes before removing from muffin or bread pans. After you have removed them from the pans, let cool for another 20 minutes.

SUPERPOWER TIP: For an extra WOW, as it pertains to a muffin, puree some strawberries and pour it on top!

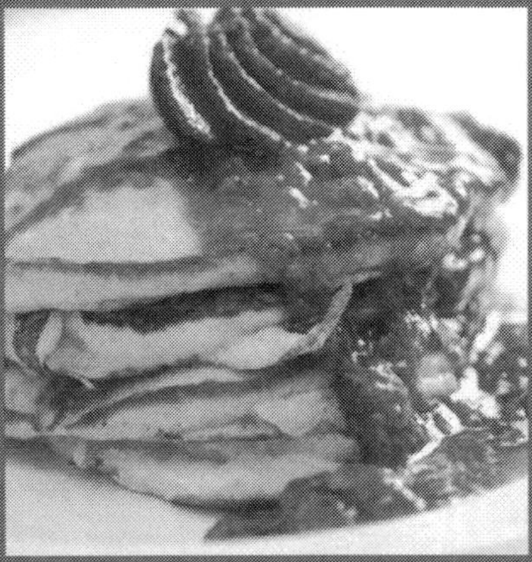

Coconut Pancakes

Coconut Protein Pancakes is one of my all-time favorites, but guess what? It's not only for breakfast; these are my go to snacks as well. Make a big batch because they store well in the fridge for a "grab and go" alternative.

Ingredients:

DF GF V

4 Eggs
1 Cup Coconut or Almond Milk
2 Tablespoons Coconut Oil (for the batter, then use extra to grease the skillet)
2 Tablespoons Honey or Maple Syrup
1/3 Cup Coconut Flour
1 teaspoon Cinnamon
1 teaspoon Vanilla
1/2 teaspoon Baking Powder
1 scoop of vanilla or coconut protein powder (I prefer to use the coconut protein powder from Superfoods Mix, look for it in the back of the book under resources)

Directions:

1. In a bowl whisk together all of the liquid ingredients, then add in the dry ingredients. You want the batter to be smooth so depending on what type of protein powder you use you may have to add a bit more of the milk. Whisk all until smooth

2. Add some coconut oil to the skillet over medium heat and spoon mixture on to skillet. Cook for about 3 minutes or once bubbles start to form and then flip and cook for another minute or so. You will end up making approx. 15 pancakes and you can top it with either maple syrup or, my all-time favorite, pureed berries. *And if you want to make it even easier....Use a waffle iron, yup they come out like waffles and are super easy to make.

SUPERPOWER TIP: Skip the maple syrup and simply puree some berries and pour that on top!

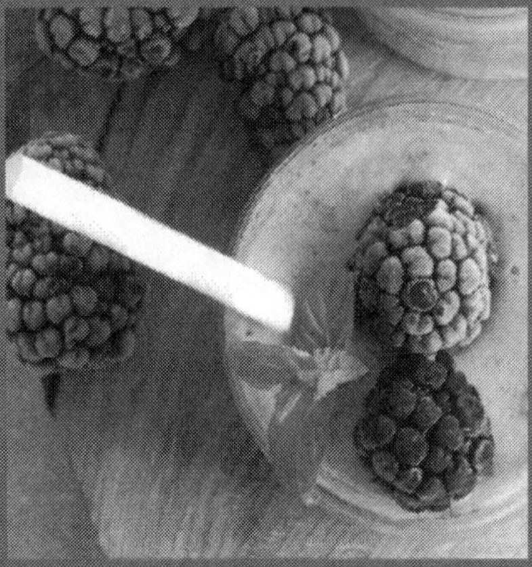

Smoothies

DF GF V 15i

Just as with any amazing recipe, you have to play with your flavors. The list below gives you the ingredients but leaves the quantities open to discussion. My recommendation is for you to start with your liquid, a little less than the size of your cup. Then, if you're a newbie, add in less than a handful of your greens and progressively add in the fruit until you reach a great taste for YOU! With time your goal is to add in more green and less fruit, but you have time, so create as you go!

Concoction	Liquid	Greens	Greens	Add Ons	Fruit	Fruit	Fruit
Immune Booster Smoothie	1 Cup Water, 1 t Lemon Juice	Collard Greens	Cucumber	Ginger	Pineapple	Mango	Banana
Blue Man Smoothie	water	Collard Greens			Blueberries Blackberries	Pear	Banana
Energy Elixir Smoothie	water	Spirulina	Kale	Cilantro	Blueberries	Goji Berries (presoaked)	Banana
Mango Mint Smoothie	water	Fresh Mint Leaves			Strawberries	Mango	Banana
Popeye's Delight	Hemp Milk	Spinach	Kale		Blueberries	Pitted Dates	Banana

Great Smoothie Additions – Protein powder (Look for my top suppliers in the back of this book), Maca (This bitter superfood helps to balance our moods and hormones, it gives us tons of vitamins and minerals, and it amps our energy, BAM!), my Nut Mix (at the end of this section), and you can also replace water for coconut water or nut milk (although hemp is one of my favorites).

SUPERPOWER TIP: When you make a bit extra, but are too full to drink it…Turn it into a frozen fruit pop (check it out in the desserts section)

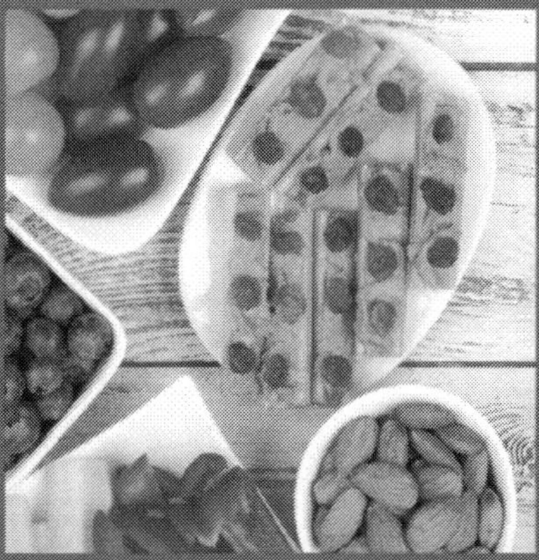

Quick Breakfast

No-Recipe Needed Quick Breakfast Suggestions

- 2 Hard or Soft Boiled Eggs
- Cut Apple with Raw Almond Butter
- Orange Slices with Raw Walnut Butter
- Egg and Avocado Wrap
- Almond Butter and Banana Wrap

Mid-Morning Snack: Again keeping with the trend of incorporating protein and a bit of fat into every meal, this snack should be just that. Here are a few suggestions to put into your arsenal of treats:

Raw Food Bars – These are "protein type bars" that have been minimally processed. I use these more as "emergency food" some of my top picks are Infinity Greens Bar, Infinity C Bar, Raw Food Bar (they have a variety of flavors), and Raw Revolution Bars (these also have a variety of flavors). Now notice how I emphasized "minimally processed" These bars are raw, they basically blend all raw ingredients, form the bar, and package it. This is a better type of food bar, it still has enzymes, and it will keep you satisfied on the run.

Fruit with Raw Nut Butter – Nut butters are so yummy, they provide quality fats and protein, the key is that they must be raw. I get pecan, almond, walnut, and cashew. Spread on or dip some fruit and you are set. I've also been known to fill the grooves of celery with almond butter and a few goji berries on top...Yum!

Raw Trail Mix – Here's the "Raw" word again, anytime you are dealing with nuts and seeds their nutrients and enzymes are at their prime, which is the true key. Once they are roasted they lose their enzymes, a few great nutrients, and the fat changes to something we really don't want in our bodies. I like to make my own; I use mulberries, goji berries, almond, cashews, coconut flakes, and any other yummy powerhouse I can find.

Get creative, I'm sure you have some favorites too, or maybe some of these have inspired a few other things not mentioned, either way it's about increasing the nutritional density and protein and you will be set. We can't have an "HANGRY" (Hungry + Angry) SuperWoman out there on the streets, nothing good will come out of it.

A great ADD-IN that you can use for any meal

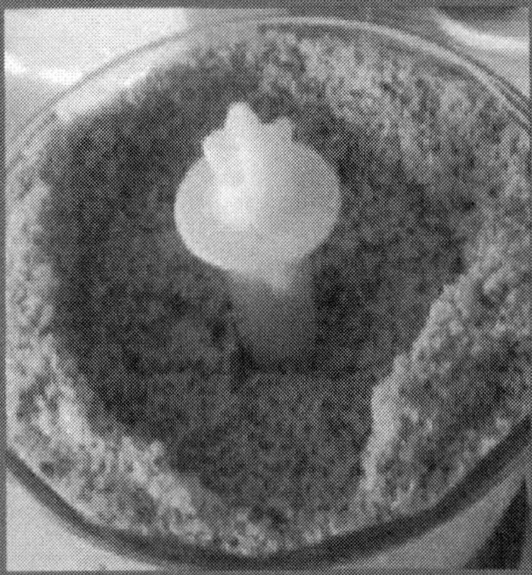

Nut Mix

Here is a great way to enhance nutrition without changing too much of the flavor. This mix is great in smoothies, salads, or anything else that needs a bit more protein.

Ideally all nuts and seeds should be organic, raw and sprouted, but at the very least make sure they are raw.

Ingredients:

Sprouted Pumpkin Seeds
Sprouted Sunflower Seeds
Hemp Seeds
Chia Seeds
Cashews
Almonds
Walnuts

Directions:

Take and pulverize them in a power blender, food processor, or coffee grinder. Blend them to a medium to fine powder and then store in an airtight container in the refrigerator.

DF GF V 15i

SUPERPOWER TIP: With time being oh so precious, make a huge batch and freeze the extra. It will last in the freezer for up to a year.

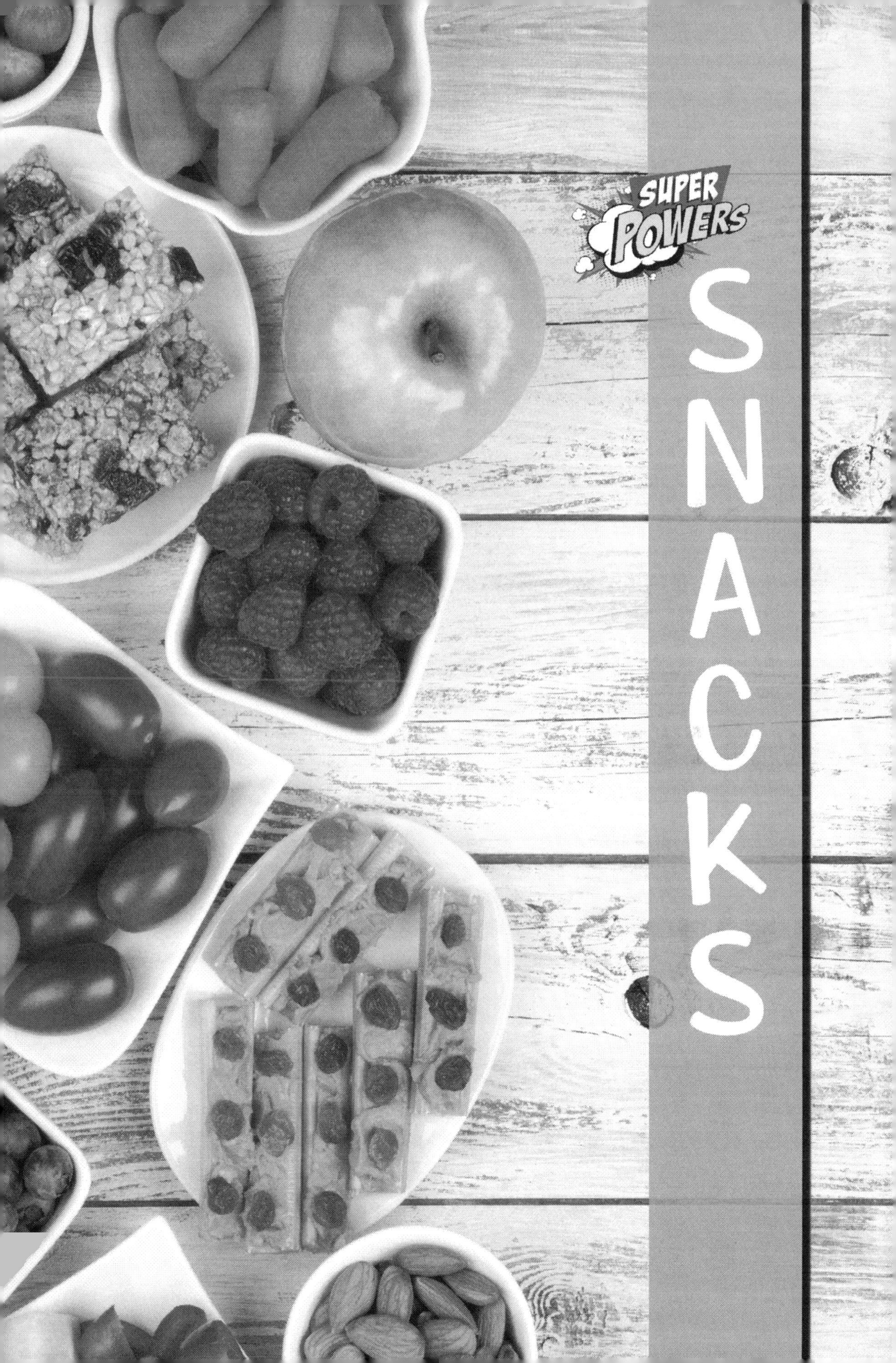
SUPER POWERS
SNACKS

Hemp Hummus

Ingredients:

1 Cup of Garbanzo Beans
1 Clove of Garlic
1 Tablespoon of Hemp Seeds
1 Tablespoon of Tahini (pureed sesame seeds)
Pinch of Salt
2-3 Tablespoon Olive Oils
And a Splash of Water
½ teaspoon Fresh Lemon Juice

Directions:

Start by blending the garlic in a high speed blender, and then add in the hemp seeds with a splash of water. Next the garbanzo beans, olive oil, tahini, salt and lemon juice. Blend until smooth – add water or additional olive oil if needed for smoothness.

DF GF V 15

SUPERPOWER TIP:
Remember, Hummus is great as a dip but it also works amazingly as a spread on a sandwich, a side for a salad, or with the Hummus Pizza as a yummy snack!

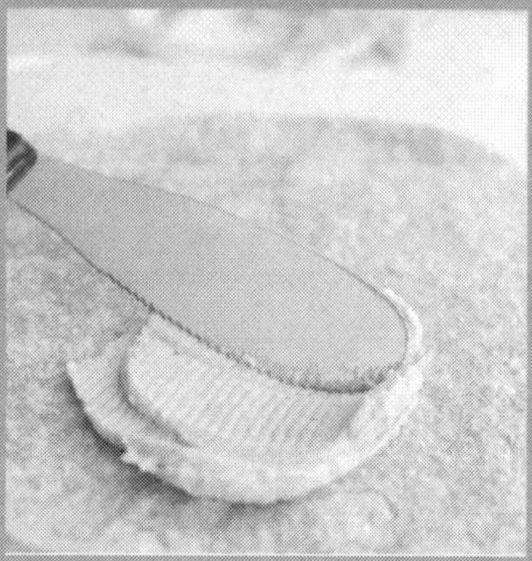

Hummus Pizza

Ingredients:

Hemp Hummus Recipe
Olive Oil
Ezekiel Wrap (this is basically a Sprouted Grain Wrap)

Directions:

Once the Hummus is ready, spread it evenly on an Ezekiel Wrap and cover with another wrap. Heat up a pan with some Olive Oil and place the "pizza" in the pan and lightly brown on both sides. Cut into diagonal slices and enjoy.

DF V 15

SUPERPOWER TIP: You can also add in sundried tomatoes, sliced veggies or a small bit of cheese to the inside with the hummus for that extra dash of flavor.

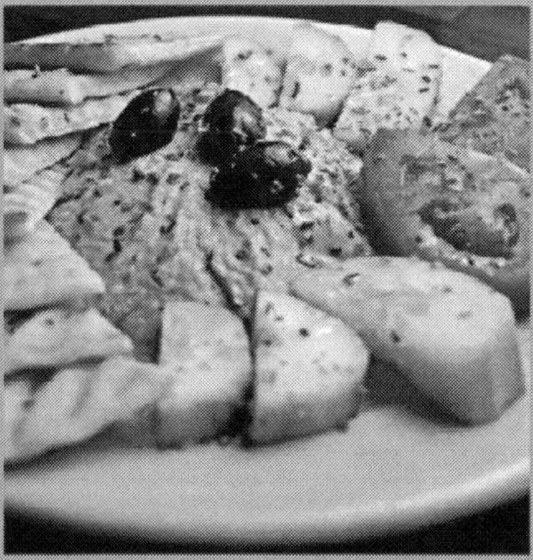

Cannellini Dip

Ingredients:

1 Cup White Kidney Beans (Cannellini Beans)
1 teaspoon fresh Lemon Juice
3 Tablespoon Olive Oil
1 clove of Garlic
1 Teaspoon Hemp Seeds
1 teaspoon chopped fresh Oregano
Pinch of salt

Directions:

Blend the garlic and hemp seeds with a dash of water in a high speed blender first, and then add in all of the additional ingredients. Blend until smooth – add water or olive oil if needed for smoothness

DF GF V 15i

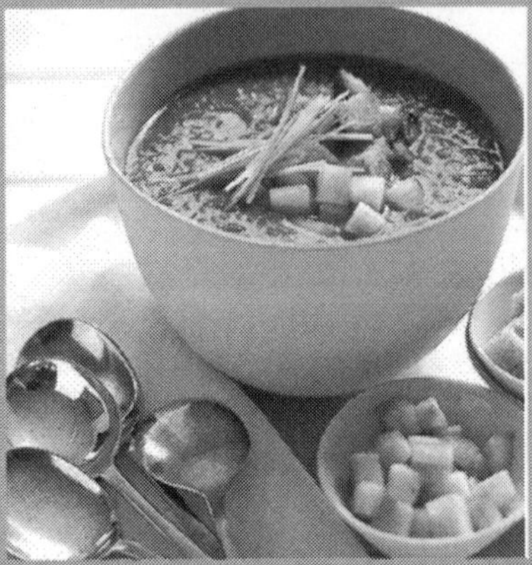

Gazpacho

Gazpacho (with a hardboiled egg)

Here is a wonderful addition to any meal and a great way to enjoy the nutrients from so many wonderful veggies. Don't be shy, think out of the box and you can easily add in a few other veggies that are not listed!!

Ingredients:

6 Large Tomatoes, fleshy and very ripe
2 Green Peppers
1 Red Pepper
1 Cucumber
1 large Onion, the heart (not the outside ring)
1 clove of Garlic
2 teaspoons Celtic or Himalayan Sea Salt
Hard Boiled Egg
Olive Oil to taste

DF GF V 15 NS

Directions:

1. Chop tomatoes, peppers, cucumber, onion and garlic. Remove the seeds from the peppers.

2. In a high speed blender, add in the veggies with a little bit of water and blend until creamy. Add cold water and mix well. And lastly add in salt and olive oil to taste.

3. A high speed blender will easily blend everything smooth, if you use a traditional blender you may want to blend again and strain to maximize smoothness (but you may end up losing some of the good stuff), also be sure to not allow a traditional blender to heat up while blending. This will allow your soup to stay enzyme rich.

4. Add more water if necessary; it must have the texture of heavy cream. Place in the refrigerator to get the desired temperature and when ready to serve sprinkle with a dash of extra virgin olive oil, mixing with a wooden spoon.

5. Serve with a garnish of diced raw cucumber, pepper onion, tomato, avocado, leeks, and a chopped hardboiled egg. Each item should be in a separate dish so that you can add them in as you like.

SUPERPOWER TIP: Pour your extra gazpacho into individual thermoses and leave them in the fridge ready to grab for at least 3 days.

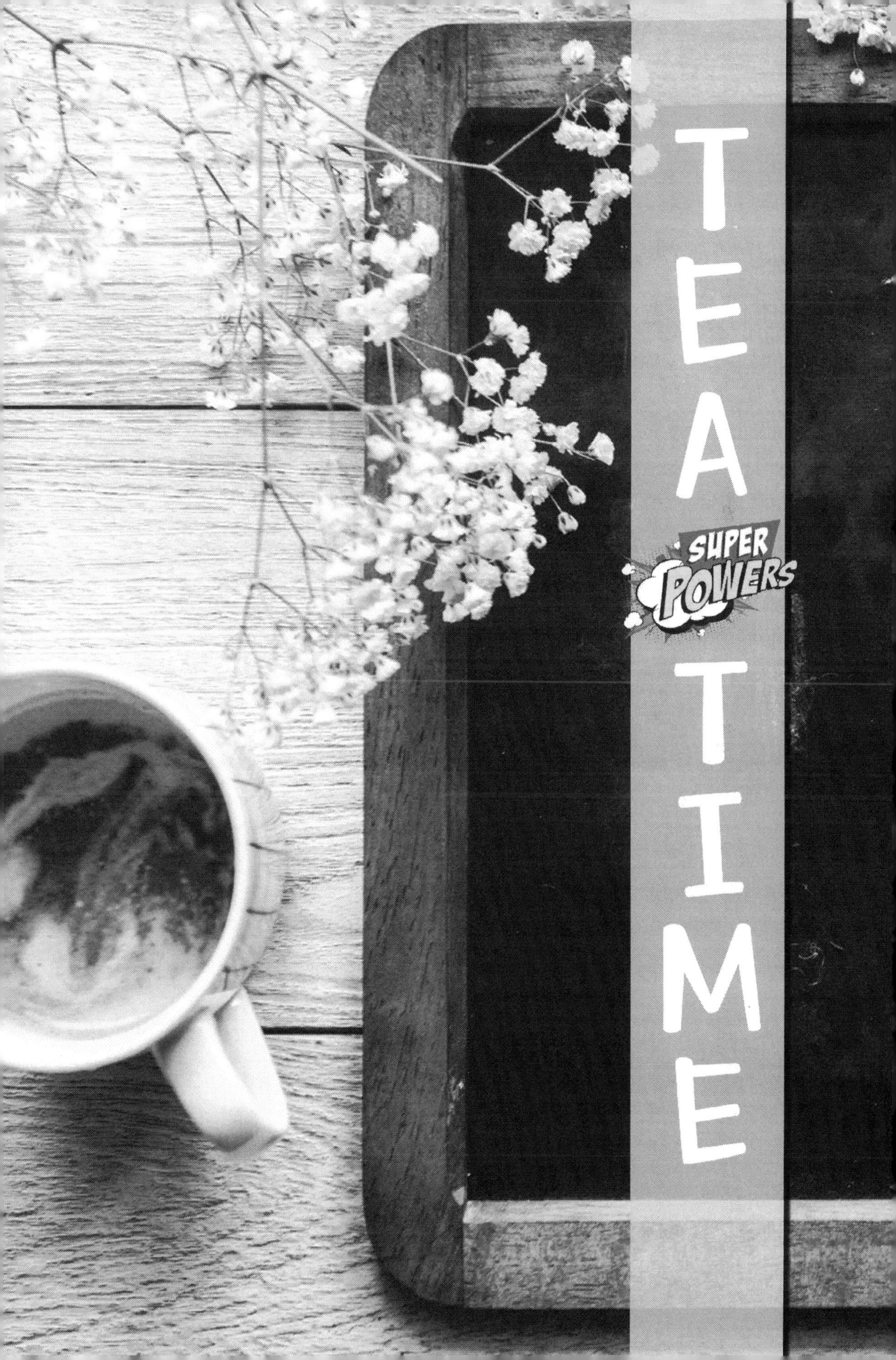
TEA
SUPER POWERS
TIME

Tea Time!

You have no idea how this makes me feel. This is my go to for adult conversation, gossip, venting, or any other excuse to meet up with my tribe. This is my time out and my recharge all combined into one, with the end result of feeling better than before. We all need that "thing" that makes us feel good and centered, this is my "thing" and I love it.

Although tea time is a ritual in my world, it also brings along a plethora of health benefits that add some extra zest into my health and into my day. Tea contains various compounds that act as antioxidants, and antioxidants are champion fighters of cell damaging free-radicals. So, all of those diseases out there can actually lose their power with these guys. Not to mention that theaninem, an amino acid found in tea, cheers on the immune system to fight infection, bacteria, and viruses. It's amazing to think that while you are sitting around the kitchen table with your besties, you can be solving world peace and bacteria all in one sip.

Top Tea Choices to Brighten your Day!

- **White Tea** is one of the premier tea selections. It goes through the least amount of processing, leaving it with the highest amount of antioxidants. This high concentration of goodness is said to aid in weight loss, as well as lowering cholesterol and fighting cancer full on. You can expect a boost of approximately 10-15 milligrams of caffeine per cup.

- **Green Tea** provides more academic accolades than any other tea. The University of Pittsburgh states that the type of antioxidants in green tea, known as polyphenols, help protect the bladder against inflammation. The University of Michigan finds the EGCG compound in green tea reduces inflammation and joint pain in rheumatoid patients. A Tufts University study stated that 1 cup of green tea provides the same antioxidant benefit as 22 vegetables, got to love it.

  There are so many more studies out there but the bottom line is that the antioxidants are outstanding and the anti-inflammatory benefits off the charts so you can't go wrong with this amazing beverage. You can expect a boost of approximately 25-30 milligrams of caffeine per cup.

- **Matcha** is also green tea but this one is a bit more special. It is harvested as the first growth of the year and pulverized so that you consume the entire leaf, providing many more antioxidant benefits, vitamin A and C, iron, and calcium, than the regular green tea varieties. Matcha is considered a "superfood" that heightens your energy, mental clarity, focus, and brings about peace, much needed for our SuperPowers. This precious gem comes in Culinary and Ceremonial varieties, providing you with a full range of quality and pricing standards. You can expect a boost of approximately 25-30 milligrams of caffeine per cup.

- **Black Tea** provides fully oxidized tea leaves, which is what gives it the darker, richer color, and the full body taste. In addition to all of the other benefits mentions, black tea has also been shown to reduce cardiovascular disease. This boost of caffeine takes it to another level, giving you 40-60 milligrams of caffeine per cup and enough energy to multitask like a true professional.

- **Oolong Tea** is created with a bit more complexity than the other tea varieties. It is withered and then rolled by hand; the leaves partially oxidize and then are fired in a pan. Oolong combines the body and richness of black tea with the fresh taste of green tea. Studies suggest that it can boost metabolism and aid in weight loss. You can expect a boost of approximately 30-50 milligrams of caffeine per cup.

- **Rooibos Tea** is a completely different animal. This tea comes from the Rooibos plant, otherwise known as Red Bush, which is grown in South Africa. This tea is totally caffeine-free but yet provides a large amount of antioxidants, vitamins, and minerals. It has been shown to decrease inflammation and alleviate such ailments such as stomach cramps. No boost of caffeine here – expect a natural type of energy with zero caffeine.

- **Herbal Teas** are typically made from an infusion of dried fruits, flowers, herbs, and spices these teas are known for their amazing smells and therapeutic properties. They come in so many flavors and varieties; they are way too many to talk about. For our purposes I have listed my top favorites but don't feel limited, the beauty of tea is to play around with flavors by combining different kinds and creating your own unique recipes. Keep in mind that many of these benefits may not help everyone, be sure to chat with your health care provider before utilizing any herbs as a treatment or therapy. Most of these provide more of a soothing type benefit so don't expect these to be "eye openers" there is no caffeine, just aromatic bliss.

- **Chamomile** – Helps to sooth the stomach and the nerves to aid in nights slumber.
- **Cinnamon** – Helps improve circulation, cold symptoms, stomach upsets and is an anti-inflammatory.
- **Echinacea** – The Immune Booster SuperHero, this one helps cold and flu symptoms and so much more.
- **Ginger** – For a "Tippy Tummy" this is your best choice, it helps with nausea, pain, inflammation, and cold symptoms.
- **Lemon** – This SuperHero of detoxification will also invigorate you for a challenging day.
- **Passionflower** – Promotes a restful sleep, lowers blood pressure, and works as a wonderful painkiller.
- **Peppermint** – Is your "go-to" for indigestion, nausea, bad breath, and cough and congestion caused by colds, yup a true mouthful!
- **Rosemary** – Is a soothing herb for headaches and fevers, and also helps with poor circulation.

Now keep in mind that all of my tea suggestions should be organic, we deserve the best of the best, so don't settle for less.

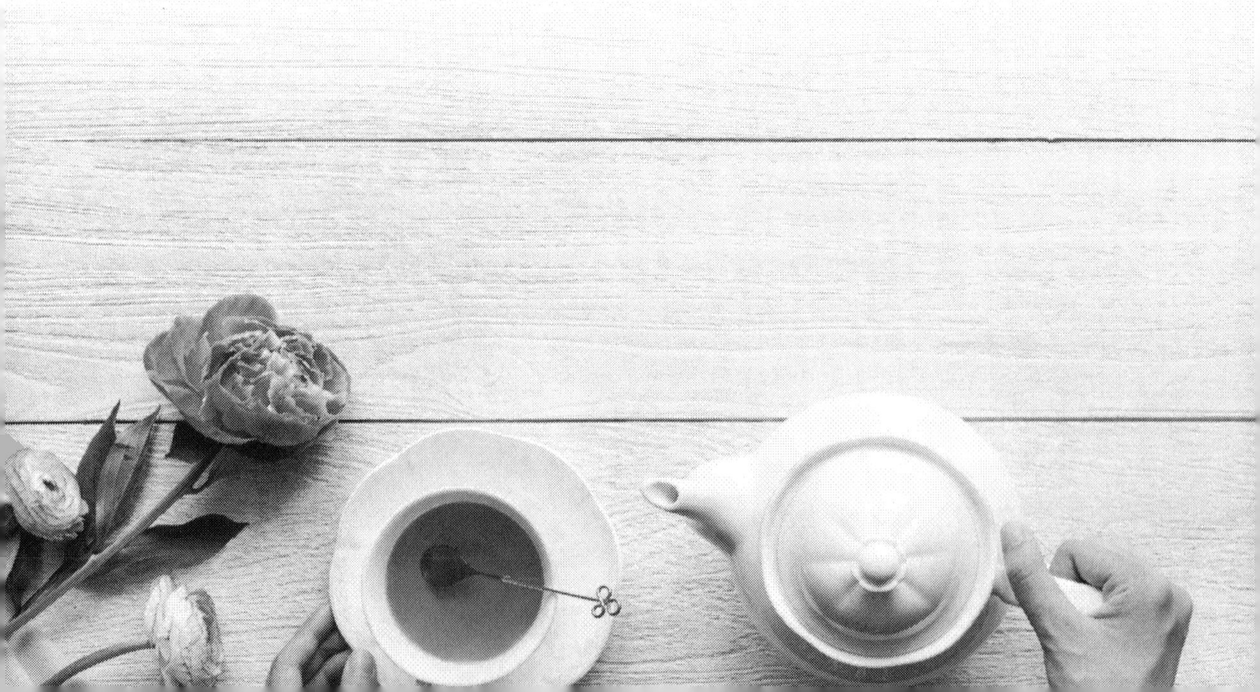

Tools of the Trade

At the end of the day, you basically need the right temperature of water and the most amazing teas in order to make yourself a cup of love and serenity. On the other hand, there are so many fun gadgets to choose from, why not use them; I have listed a few in my order of preference:

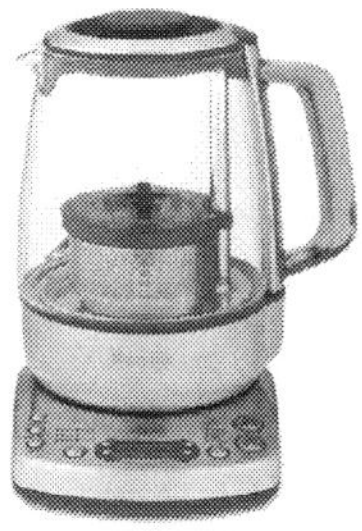

#1 I live for my Breville One-Touch Tea Maker (do you think Breville will send me a new one for this marketing plug?). It's a bit expensive but I use it EVERYDAY, sometimes 2-3 times a day, so it is totally worth it. I can even set it to have my tea made to perfection when I get out of bed. For years I only thought coffee makers did that, who knew. I have all of my teas in jars and I sit in front of my tea maker creating new combinations like a mad scientist.

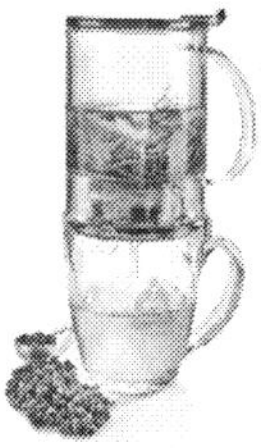

#2 Loose Leaf Tea Infusers - They have some that look like a tea cup with a handle and then you simply set it on top of your mug and your tea drips right on in. Then there are the insulated bottles that have the infuser built in so that you can take it on the go. And last but not least, you have the tea pot that will infuse the tea as well.

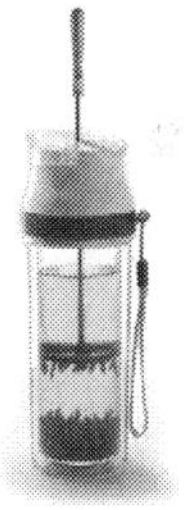

#3 Tea Bag Replacements – There are a wide variety of tea balls or you have tea bags that you can simply fill up yourself (this one is a great project for the kids or a coworker that needs something to do).

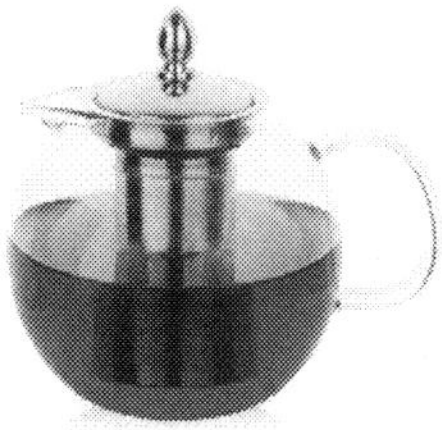

#4 Tea Bags – Yup this one is last, you can still make some good combinations with these, they are just not as fun.

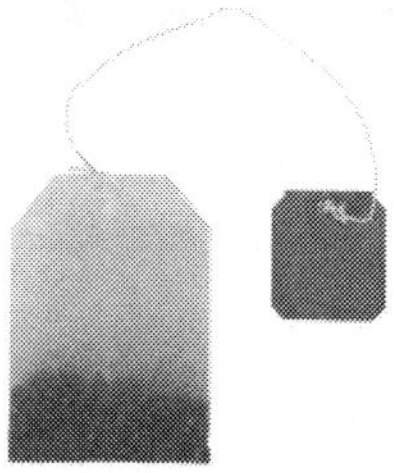

Brewing Instructions

Not every tea brews the same, you want to preserve it benefits and enhance its many flavors. When creating your recipe a good standard guideline is one rounded teaspoon per eight oz. cup. This refers to a measuring teaspoon, not the teaspoon in your silverware set which is usually much larger than a true measuring teaspoon.

- **White Teas** should be steeped anywhere from 175 – 185 degrees, when you see the very first hint of steam. White teas are steeped 3-4 minutes, although some can be steeped much longer with tasty results.

- **Green Teas** should be made with slightly cooler water, between 165 and 180 degrees. Green teas are steeped for much less time, 2-3 minutes. Stronger ones as little as 1 minute or to taste.

- **Black Tea** generally should be made with water at a full, rolling boil, 212 degrees. Black teas steep 3-5 minutes. Darjeeling's are the exceptions; they should be steeped 2-3 minutes.

- **Oolong Tea** should be made with water a little bit below boiling, between 185 and 200 degrees. Oolong teas vary dramatically and you need to experiment or follow the suggested steeping instructions on the bag. Many oolongs are perfect at 3-4 minutes; some need 6-8 minutes. It is common to warm oolong leaves first in order to achieve full flavor or fragrance. To do this pour hot water (200 degrees) over tealeaves, pour out immediately and discard the water. Now the tea is ready for steeping.

The rule with most rooibos and herbal teas is to "steep longer for stronger".

- **Herbal Teas** should typically be made with boiling water, 212 degrees.

- **Rooibos** should typically be made with boiling water, 212 degrees. Rooibos should be steeped a minimum of 4-6 minutes, some for up to 10 minutes.

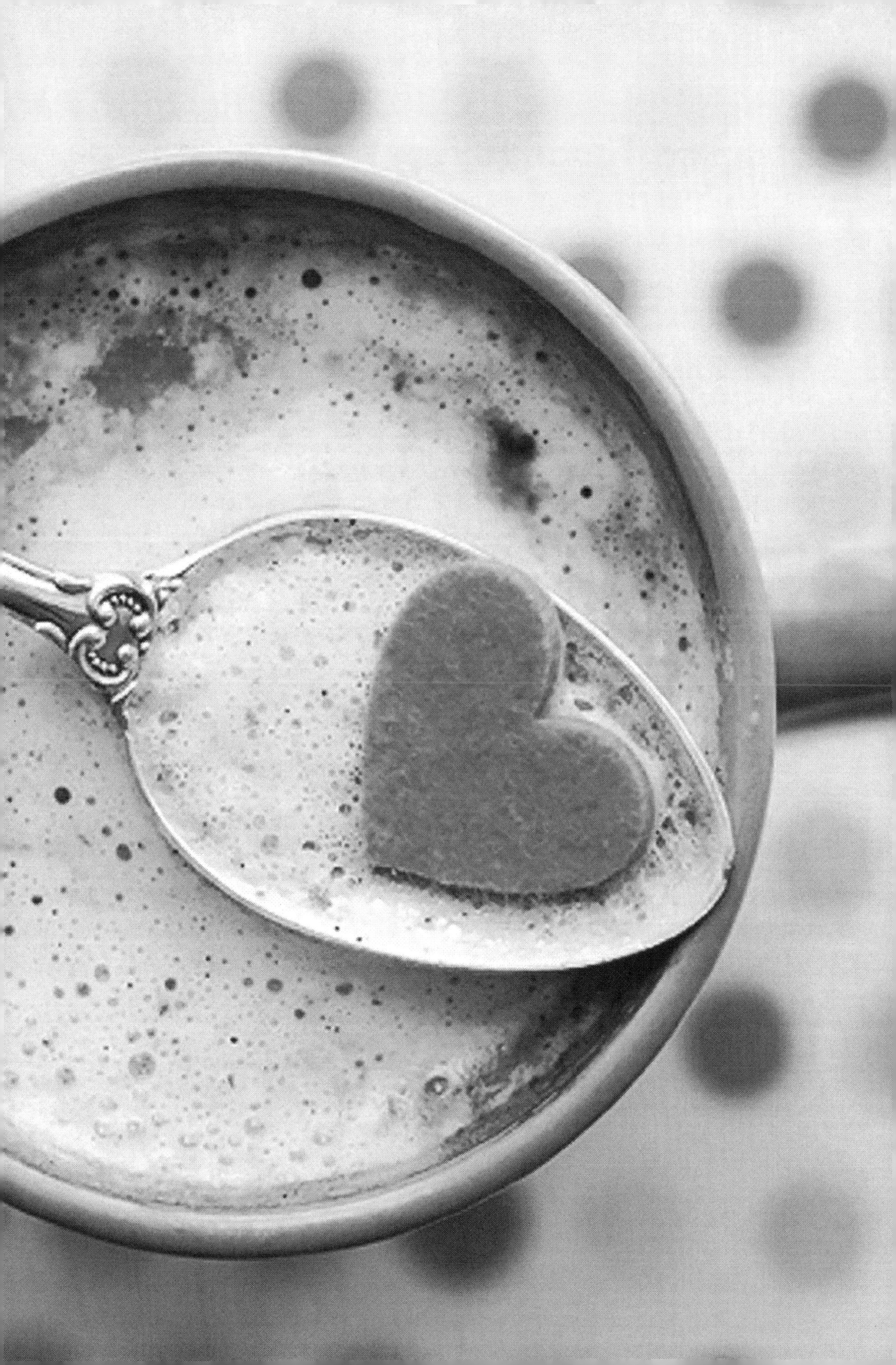

It's Tea Time!! Recipes for your tribe

Brew and Enjoy!

My all-time favorite tea is a well brewed Chai Latte, can I tell you...

I love Chai, I love Chai, I love Chai, I Love Chai!

So what is chai? "Chai" is the Hindi word for "tea," which was derived from "cha," which is the Chinese word for "tea." So what is chai tea? It's essentially "tea tea" that is made customarily in India, where it's commonly called masala chai. They combine a mix of spices and herbs to create the warm and spicy flavor that make chai so amazing.

Coconut Chai

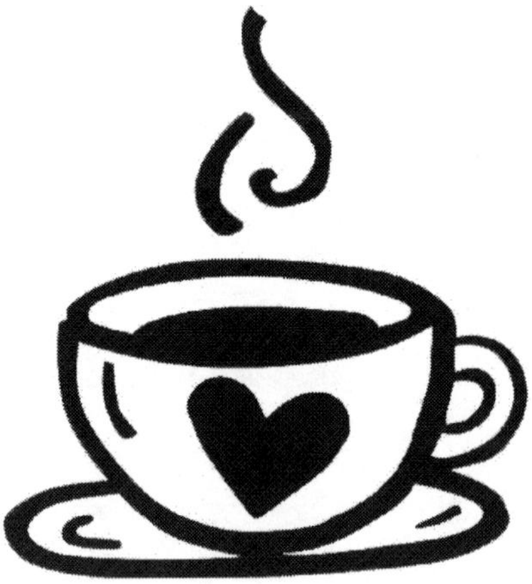

Ingredients:

2 Cup Coconut Milk
1 Date, pitted
½–1 Tablespoon Honey or Maple Syrup
½ teaspoon Cinnamon
⅛ teaspoon Ginger
⅛ teaspoon Cardamom
⅛ teaspoon Nutmeg
⅛ teaspoon ground Cloves
1 teaspoon unsweetened shredded Coconut

Directions:

Warm the coconut milk over medium heat until hot..
Next, place the hot milk into a high speed blender and add in the remaining ingredients.
Blend until well combined and smooth.
Pour and enjoy!

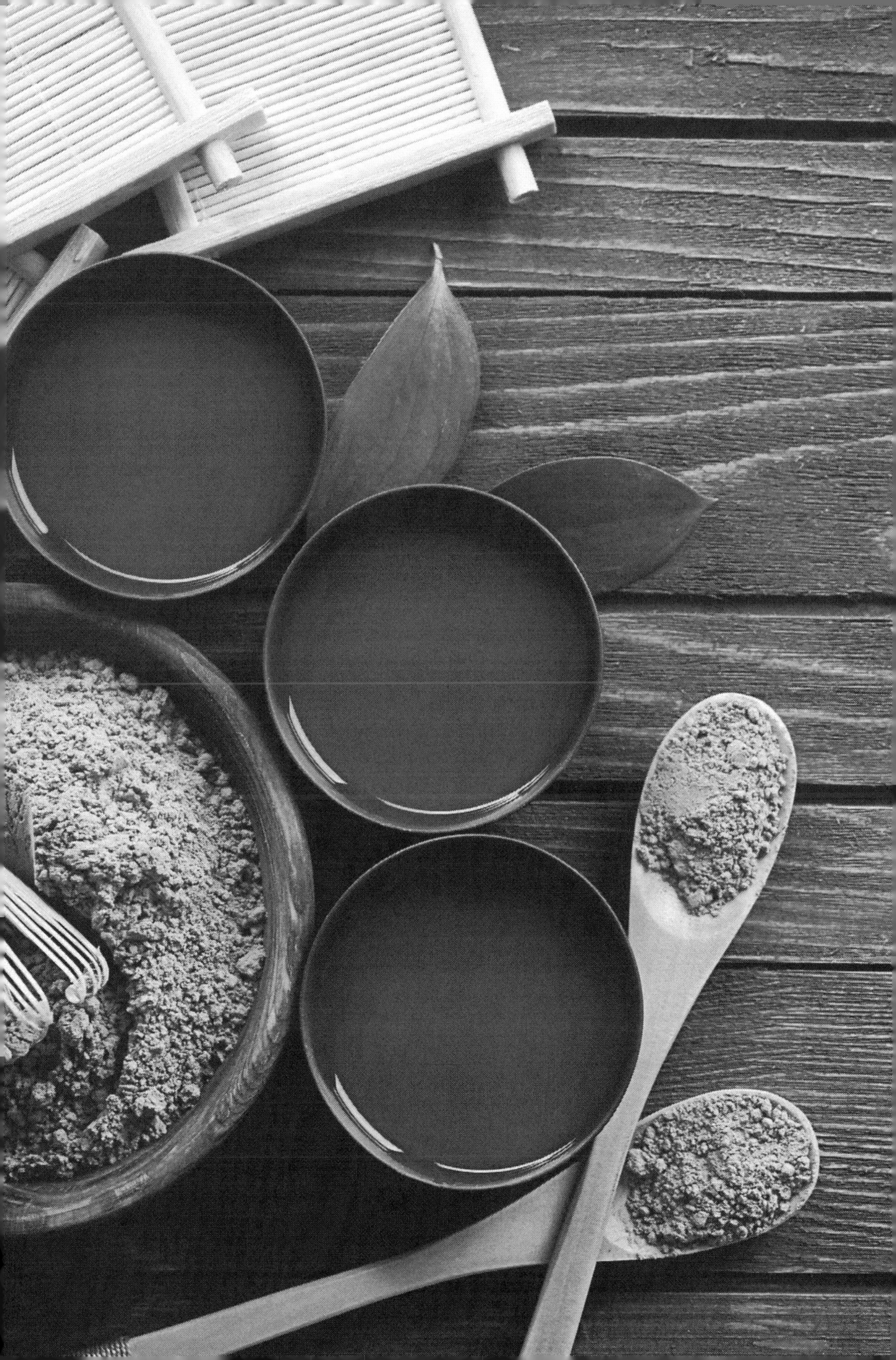

Chocolate Matcha Latte

Ingredients:

2 teaspoon Matcha and 3 oz. Hot Water
1T organic Dark Chocolate Chips
1 tsp Coconut Oil or MCT Oil
1–2 teaspoon organic raw Honey
1 ½ Cup Hemp Milk

Directions:

Whisk matcha tea in a bowl with the water. In a separate pan, warm hemp milk on medium heat over the stove and add chocolate bits, slowly stirring until chocolate completely melts. Next combine hot chocolate, honey, oil, and matcha and top with a dash of cinnamon.

Now, this recipe is amazing when you whisk your matcha to perfection, but for those occasional moments when you *NEED* your matcha *NOW*, pull out the high speed blender and make it happen!

Adita's Matcha Latte

Ingredients:

1½ Cup Hemp or Coconut Milk
1 teaspoon Ceremonial-Grade Matcha
1 teaspoon Coconut Oil or MCT Oil
1–2 teaspoon organic raw Honey

Directions:

In a teakettle or small pot, warm the milk. In a blender, add the milk and all the other ingredients. Blend in a high speed blender until smooth. Top with cinnamon, serve and enjoy!

Just a side note – true Ceremonial tea is properly whisked to perfection, I started this way but my need for my matcha and my lack of time sent me down the rabbit hole looking for my blender.

Pumpkin Spiced Matcha

Ingredients:

1 Tablespoon Pumpkin Pie Spice (cinnamon, cloves, nutmeg, ginger)
1 Cup boiled Water, cooled to about 74 degrees
2 teaspoon Honey
1 teaspoon Matcha Green Tea Powder
1 Tablespoon Pumpkin Purée (look at the ingredients – nothing more than pumpkin!)
1 Cup Coconut Milk

Directions:

In a small sauce pan, place water to boil. Once boiled, remove from heat and allow to cool to 74 degrees.

Place matcha green tea into a mixing bowl and add in a small amount of the 74 degree water. Whisk the water and tea vigorously until bubbles form. Slowly pour the rest of the water over the Matcha, and stir it until it's fully combined and turns a dark green color.

At the same time, heat up the milk, pumpkin pie spice, pumpkin purée, and honey. Stir to combine, then whip over medium heat until frothy. (Or, if you have a milk frother, you can simply use that.) Then pour with pleasure over your Matcha and sprinkle some extra cinnamon on top for good merits

The Reserve

Brew in large batches to use throughout the week

Ginger Chai Reserve

This tea recipe is considered a *reserve* because you can easily make the tea with no milk and store it in the refrigerator for up to a month. During this time the flavors will deepen and then you can quickly take out a cup, add in the milk, and boil to perfection on a spare of the moment.

Ingredients:

1 Tablespoon Fennel Seed
6 Green Cardamom Pods
14 whole Cloves
2 Cinnamon Stick
1 (1/4-inch) piece Ginger Root, peeled and thinly sliced
6 Black Peppercorns
7 Cup Water
2 Tablespoon Black Tea
2 Tablespoon organic Honey or to taste

Directions:

Boil for 5 minutes, from here you can store it for future use or serve. One quick note – if you enjoy strong flavors as I do, you may want to leave all of the spices soaking in the stored tea for the first week and then filter them out before use, just a thought.

Now, when you are ready to serve add in the milk...
1 C Hemp Milk (heated at medium heat until hot)

If you are storing the brewed tea and then making your tea on the spot, simply boil with the milk for a few minutes or until it reaches a temperature that you enjoy.

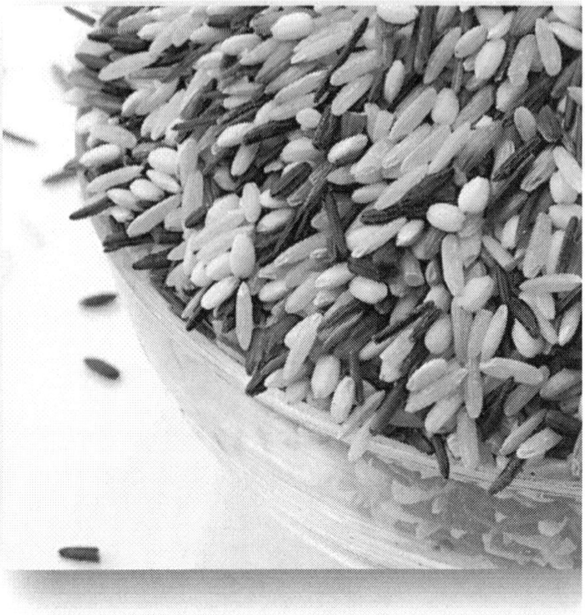

My Favorite Dry Mix Recipes

These recipes are designed to make you big batches of yummy dry blends that you can use to make that great cup of tea, on demand, at a later date. Remember to keep all of your ingredients organic. These are fun tea blends, you can also add in your favorite nut milk and honey or drink it straight up, *whatever the mood calls for.*

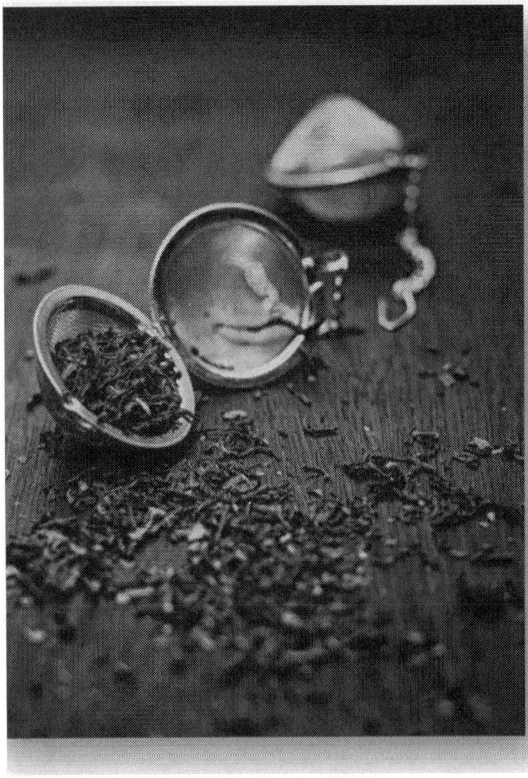

Toasted Rice Green Tea

Ok, so this one requires a bit of work but it is totally worth the effort and you can toast a bit more for the other recipes in this section as well. In my world, I like to make a huge batch so that I have it easily available in times of need.

Ingredients:

2 Cup loose Green Tea
1 Cup Wild Rice, toasted
1 Cup Jasmine Rice, toasted

Directions:

Remember you can play with the measurements depending on how big a batch you want to make.

In a dry and shallow pan, combine the Wild Rice and Jasmine Rice. There is no oil needed here, simply place your heat at a low temperature and toast the rice stirring it constantly with a wood spoon to keep the rice from burning. After it is toasted, and smelling oh so yummy, let it sit until completely cooled. This may take an hour or so.

Next, combine the cooled rice with the tea and stir until combined. Then make yourself a great cup of tea and store the rest in an airtight container for future use.

Morning Wake-Up Call

You can use your Toasted Rice Green Tea Recipe and then add in the black tea and cacao nibs or make the entire thing from scratch, up to you.

Ingredients:

½ - 1 Cup loose Black Tea
1 Cup loose Green Tea
1 Cup Wild Rice, toasted
1 Cup Jasmine Rice, toasted
1 Cup Cacao Nibs

Directions:

In a dry and shallow pan, combine the wild rice and jasmine rice. There is no oil needed here, simply place your heat at a low temperature and toast the rice stirring it constantly with a wood spoon to keep the rice from burning. After it is toasted, and smelling yummy, let it sit until completely cooled. This may take an hour or so.

Next, combine the cooled rice with the tea and stir until completely combined. Then make yourself a great cup of tea and store the rest in an airtight container for future use.

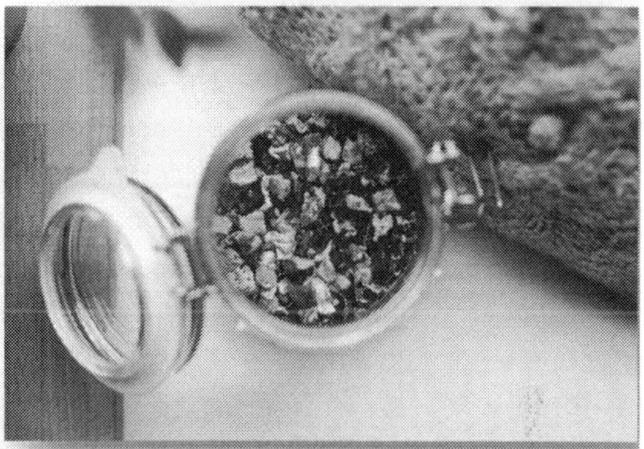

Morning Chai with a Twist

Ingredients:

½ Cup Black Peppercorn
½ Cup dry Ginger Root
6 Cinnamon Sticks
2 Tablespoon dry Burdock Root
¼ Cup dry Elderberry

¼ Cup Dry Goji Berry
2 Tablespoon Fennel Seed
2 Tablespoon Cardamom Seeds
3 Tablespoon Green Cardamom Pods
10 Cloves
½ Cup Holy Basil (so good for stress!)
¼ Cup Cacao Nibs
½ Cup loose Green Tea (or do a combination of both black and green tea for an extra "something, something")
2 Vanilla Bean pods (chopped to approx. 1/8")
15 strands Saffron

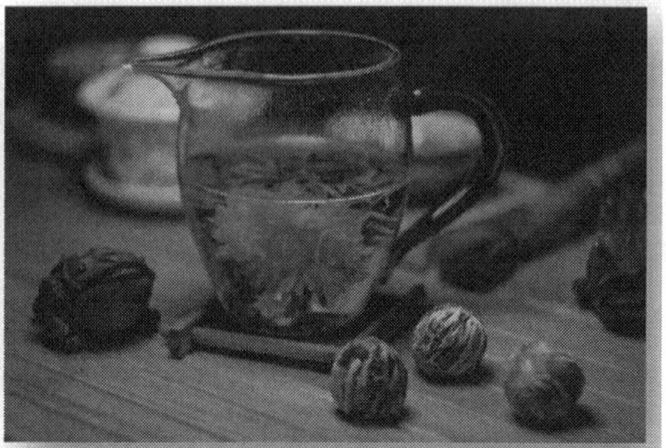

Directions:

Measure and combine all of the ingredients in a large bowl, then stir gently with a spoon until mixed well. Next, take the saffron between your fingers and crush it over the blend. Give it one more stir to make sure it is all well combined. Then make yourself a great cup of tea and store the rest in an airtight container for future use.

I don't know about you but I am all about wonderful smells, this is your tea, so smell it and tweak the recipe accordingly until you get that wonderful aroma that inspires you to make that cup of tea NOW.

Serenity Tea

Ingredients:

1 Cup Chamomile
½ Cup Dandelion Root
½ Cup Chrysanthemum
1 Cup Goji Berry
1 Cup Green Tea
1/8 Cup dried Mint Leaf
½ Cup Lemongrass
½ Cup Holy Basil
3-4 Vanilla Bean Pods (chopped to approx. 1/8")

Directions:

Mix all of the ingredients in a large bowl and store in an airtight container for future use, but first make yourself a cup so that you can bask in the glory.

SUPERPOWER TIP: Remember there is no right, or wrong way to prepare tea drinks. Try different ratios and ingredients until you get it just the way you like it. I go by the smell, if it smells inviting…It's a winner.

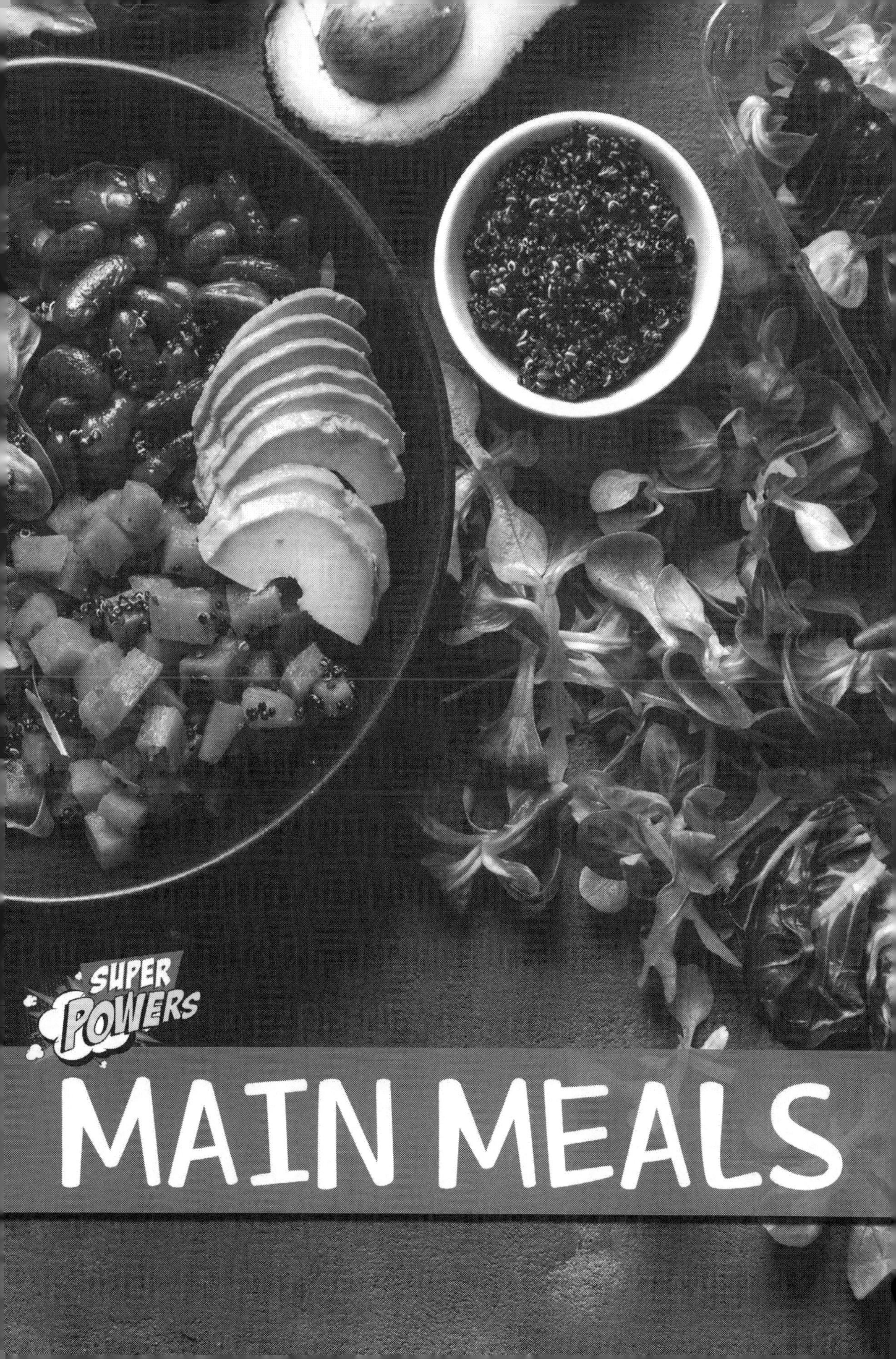

SUPER POWERS

MAIN MEALS

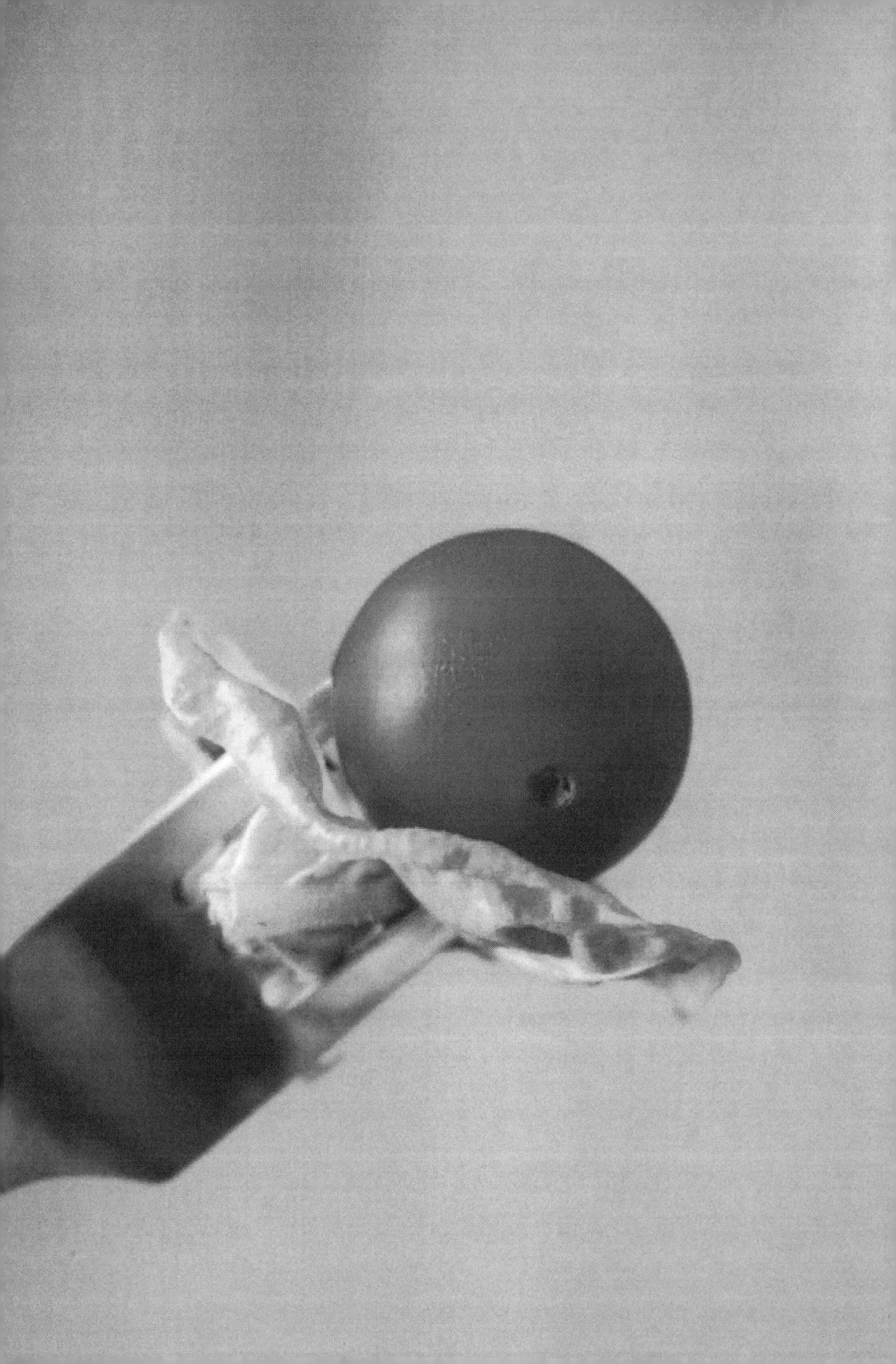

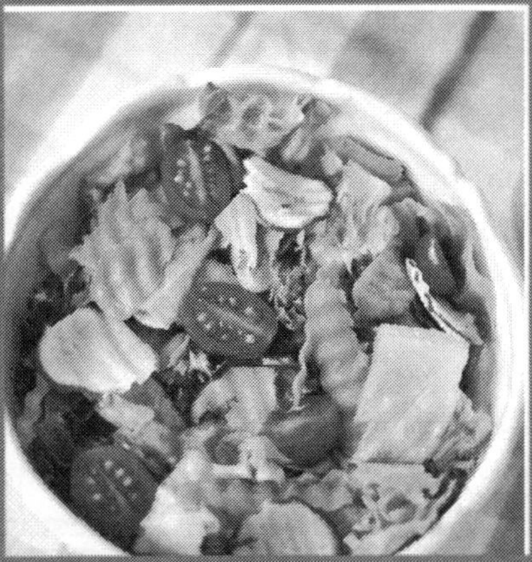

Basic Salad

Ingredients:

Use Kitchen Scissors to easily chop

Greens
Spinach
Collard Greens
Romaine
Tomatoes
Carrots
Avocado
Nut Mix
Cold Pressed Olive Oil

Directions:

Hopefully you have pre chopped most of your veggies, if not get to chopping! Then use your kitchen scissors to cut up your greens into small, bite size, bits. From here you dress up your salad with nut mix, and olive oil or any other dressing combination that is not creamy and thick and ooey and gooey. Next, don't forget your protein, you can add in any leftovers you have around! – Chicken, meat or even a hardboiled egg, if that doesn't work add in extra nut mix or some beans.

DF GF V 15i NS

SUPERPOWER TIP: Sitting down to lunch in my world is a luxury that I haven't partaken in in quite a while. My typical food choices that I can grab and go include Part Two of my morning smoothie, hummus and veggies to dip, or a quick salad from my pre-prepped veggie assortment.

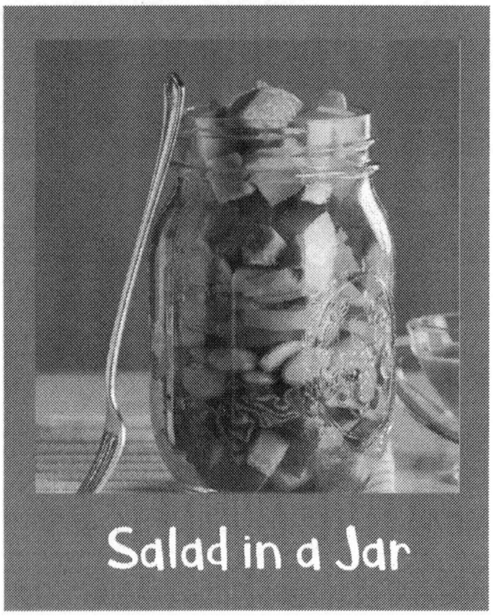

This is so very ingenious but there is a Fine Art to Packing the Perfect Jar!

The easiest jars to use are the quart-size jars with wide-mouth lids, these are simple to fill and eat out of. Next for this to really work you need to make sure they can be sealed and kept upright.

1. Start with salad dressing. Since you keep the jar upright, the salad dressing will stay at the bottom and separated from your veggies.

2. Next up are your Veggies. Place your harder veggies like carrots, radishes, and onions. These will still stay crisp even if they mix with the dressing. Then go for anything else like bell peppers, chopped cucumbers, cherry tomatoes, and any beans you would like to add in.

3. Layers of greens. This should take up at least half the jar. Wash your leafy greens and let them dry completely (you may want to use a paper towel for this one), then use your kitchen scissors and slice them up for your jar.

4. Last up...Protein. Here you can add in sliced up chicken or meat, these will help weigh everything down in the jar so you can add even more to your jar. At this point you can also add avocado, nut mix or individual nuts or seeds to top it off. Your meat choice and/or avocado should be added the day you are eating your jar, this way the other ingredients remain as fresh as possible.

5. Time to Enjoy! When you're ready, just shake it up or dump it out into a bowl – whichever is the easiest.

DF GF V 15i NS

SUPERPOWER TIP: A well-organized jar can last you 3 days in the fridge.

Storage Suggestions to keep your Veggies Fresh and Convenient

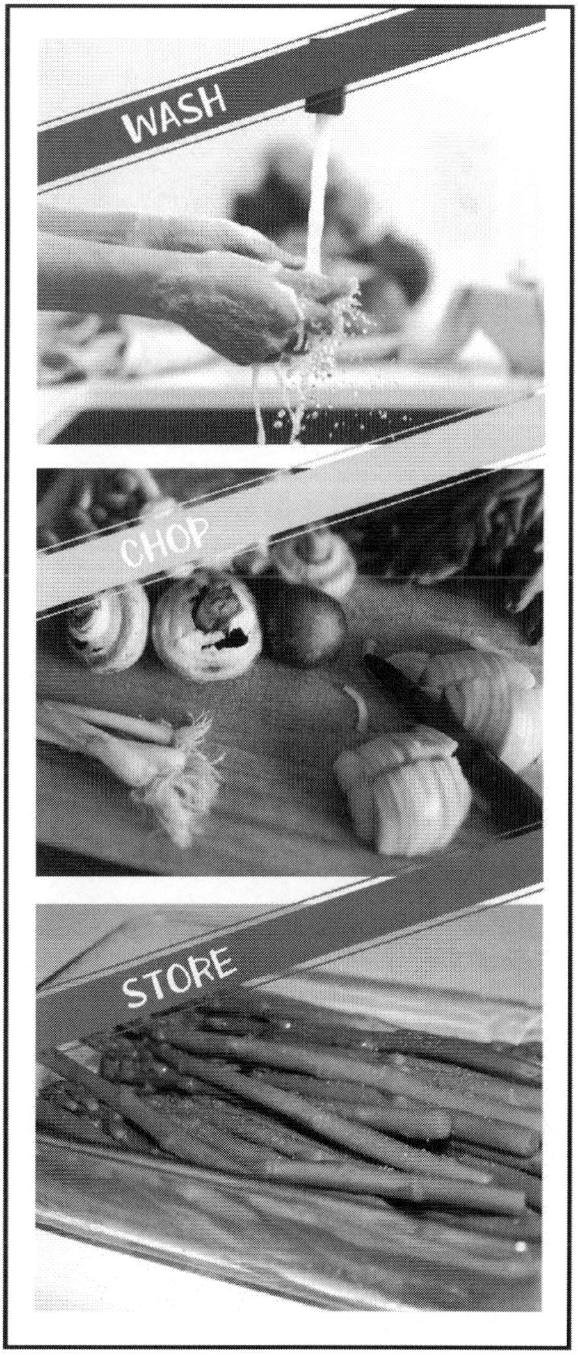

First wash your veggies and allow them to completely dry before chopping and storing. Now with all of your harder type veggies you can easily chop and store them in an airtight container for up to 5 days. Tomatoes can be chopped and placed in an airtight container for up to 3 days. Your leafy greens should not be washed until you are about to use them, you should, however, store your larger leafs by placing the stems in a glass of water with the leaves covered by a plastic bag. This will keep them fresh for at least a week. For avocados, keep them on the counter if they are hard, once they are soft store in the refrigerator.

Ideally you can create a shelf in your refrigerator that holds all of your veggie containers so that you can easily take a spoonful out for any recipe you have in mind! The objective is to keep things simple, take a day a week for food prep, it may sound like extras work but it will save you and your eating habits on a day to day basis.

Avocado Chicken Salad Wrap

Ingredients: DF NS

Cooked Organic Chicken
Avocado
Celtic Sea Salt
Olive Oil
Ezekiel Wrap

Directions:

Shred the chicken and combine it with mashed avocado (the all-time best substitute for mayo!). Next, place the mixture inside an ezekiel wrap. Add a drizzle of olive oil and a dash of celtic sea salt to taste. For an added nutritional boost, that does not change the flavor, add in some Hemp Seeds.

SUPERPOWER TIP: As a Gluten Free alternative – Replace the wrap with a giant lettuce or collard green leaf!

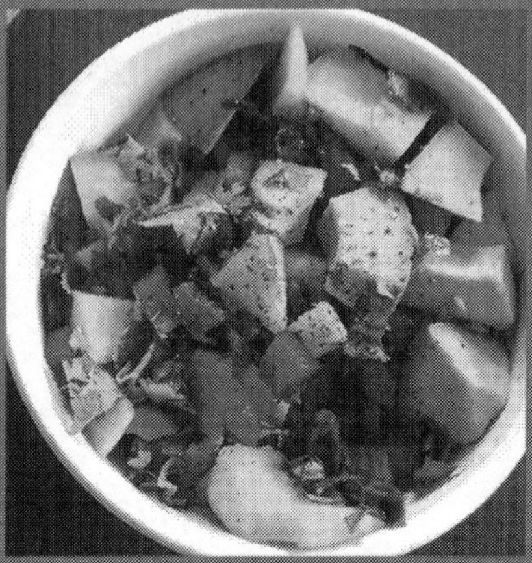

Mango Avocado

Ingredients:

Serves 4
1 large Cucumber, cubed (1/4 inch)
1 Cup Cherry Tomatoes, halved
½ Cup chopped Green Beans
½ Cup Bean Sprouts
1 medium Mango, peeled and sliced
1 medium Avocado, peeled and sliced
¼ Cup finely chopped Mint

Directions: Mix and add in dressing

Dressing:
1/3 Cup Rice Vinegar
2 Tablespoons Lime Juice
2 Chilies, minces
1 teaspoon Honey

DF GF V 15

Quinoa Salad

Ingredients:

Cooked Quinoa
Japanese Peppers
Yellow Bell Pepper
Sundried Tomatoes in Olive Oil
White Beans
Baby Tomatoes
Cold Pressed Olive Oil
Celtic or Himalayan Sea Salt

Directions:

Chop your veggies and mix it all up. Play with your flavors and create the right amounts of each ingredient to **tantalize your taste buds**, Enjoy!

DF GF V 15 NS

SUPERPOWER TIP: On your Food-Prep days, cook up plain quinoa, this stays good in the fridge for up to 5 days and then you can easily add it into a meal, "just a thought".

Almond Leek Soup

Ingredients:

1 Cup blanched Almonds
6 Cups Chicken or Vegetable Broth
2 Cups coarse chopped Celery
1 medium coarse chopped Leek, white parts only
1 Tablespoon Olive Oil
Salt and Pepper, to taste

Directions:

Simmer almonds in broth until soft, about 30 minutes. Next, sauté the leeks and the celery until they are soft. Add sautéed vegetables to almonds and broth. Simmer until soft, about 15 minutes and let cool for 10-15 minutes or until temperature is 120F. Then blend with a high powered blender until smooth and Enjoy!

DF GF V NS

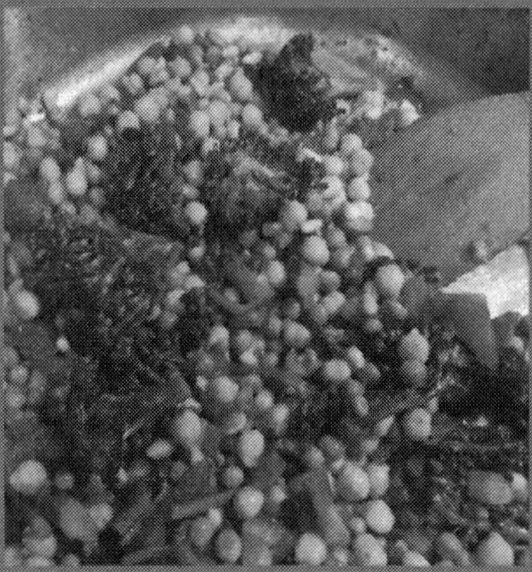

Quinoa Veggie Blend

This one gives you a full meal in minutes. Enjoy a quick blend of quinoa and vegetables to provide you with amazing nutrients and protein.

Ingredients:

1 Cup cooked Quinoa
Extra Virgin Olive Oil
2 Cloves Garlic, finely chopped
1/4 Cup Pine Nuts
1 1/2 Cups chopped Broccoli
1 chopped Red Pepper
1 Cup cooked White Beans
1 large chopped Tomato
Celtic Sea Salt
Water

Directions: DF GF V NS

In a medium sauté pan heat the olive oil and garlic at a medium heat, once garlic starts to brown add in the broccoli. Throw in a dash of water and allow the broccoli to turn a bright green, then add in the white beans and red peppers, let this cook for about five minutes. Finally add in the tomatoes and season with a bit of salt to taste. Serve over a bed of quinoa and enjoy!

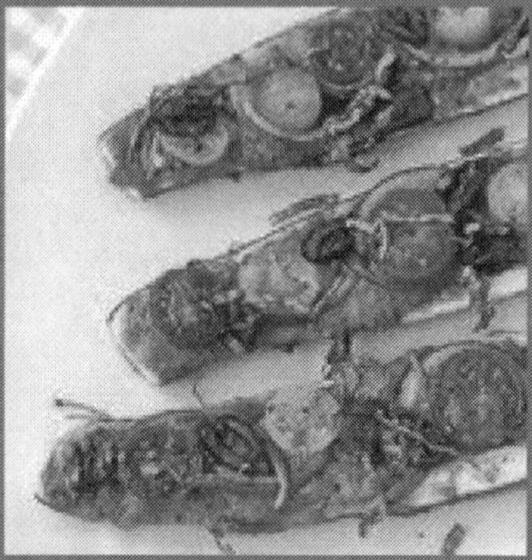

Zucchini Pizza

Ingredients:

4 large Zucchini
2 finely chopped large Tomatoes
5 finely chopped Sun-dried Tomatoes
1/2 Tablespoon fresh Garlic
1/4 teaspoon Oregano
1/4 teaspoon Dried Basil or 12 large fresh Basil Leaves
Salt to taste
*For the Cheese Lovers - Grated Fresh Parmigiano Cheese

Directions:

1. On the stove top sauté the garlic, tomatoes, sun-dried tomatoes, oregano, and dried basil (if you opt for fresh leaves - leave these for right before putting on the cheese). Sauté for a couple of minutes

2. Cut the Zucchini in half-length wise, place in a roasting pan with the cut side up. Spread the tops with the sautéed mixture and add the cheese (these can be made with or without cheese)

3. Place in the oven at 350 for about 35 minutes and Enjoy!!

DF GF V NS

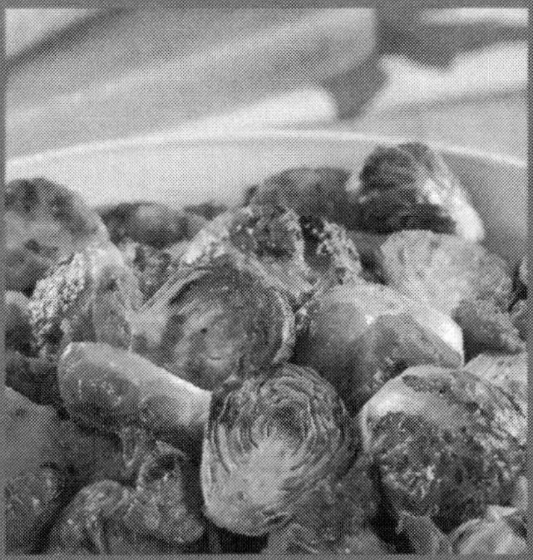
Brussel Sprouts

Roasted Brussel Sprouts

Ingredients:

1 ½ lbs. of Brussel Sprouts (ends cut with any yellow leaves removed)
1 Tablespoon of Maple Syrup
3 Tablespoons of Olive Oil
2 Tablespoons chopped Garlic
1 teaspoon Celtic Sea Salt
4 Tablespoons of chopped Sundried Tomatoes (the ones that come in Olive Oil)

Directions:

Preheat oven to 450 degrees. Chop the Brussel sprouts into quarters, and then add in the maple syrup, olive oil, garlic, and salt and mix up well. Next, place those ingredients spread out into a baking dish and put into a preheated oven for 35 minutes. At the 35 minute mark, mix everything up again and add in the sundried tomatoes, place back into oven for 10 minutes. You want everything dark and crispy! As an added alternative I add in cooked Cannellini Beans with the sundried tomatoes and then serve it on a bed of quinoa.

DF GF V NS

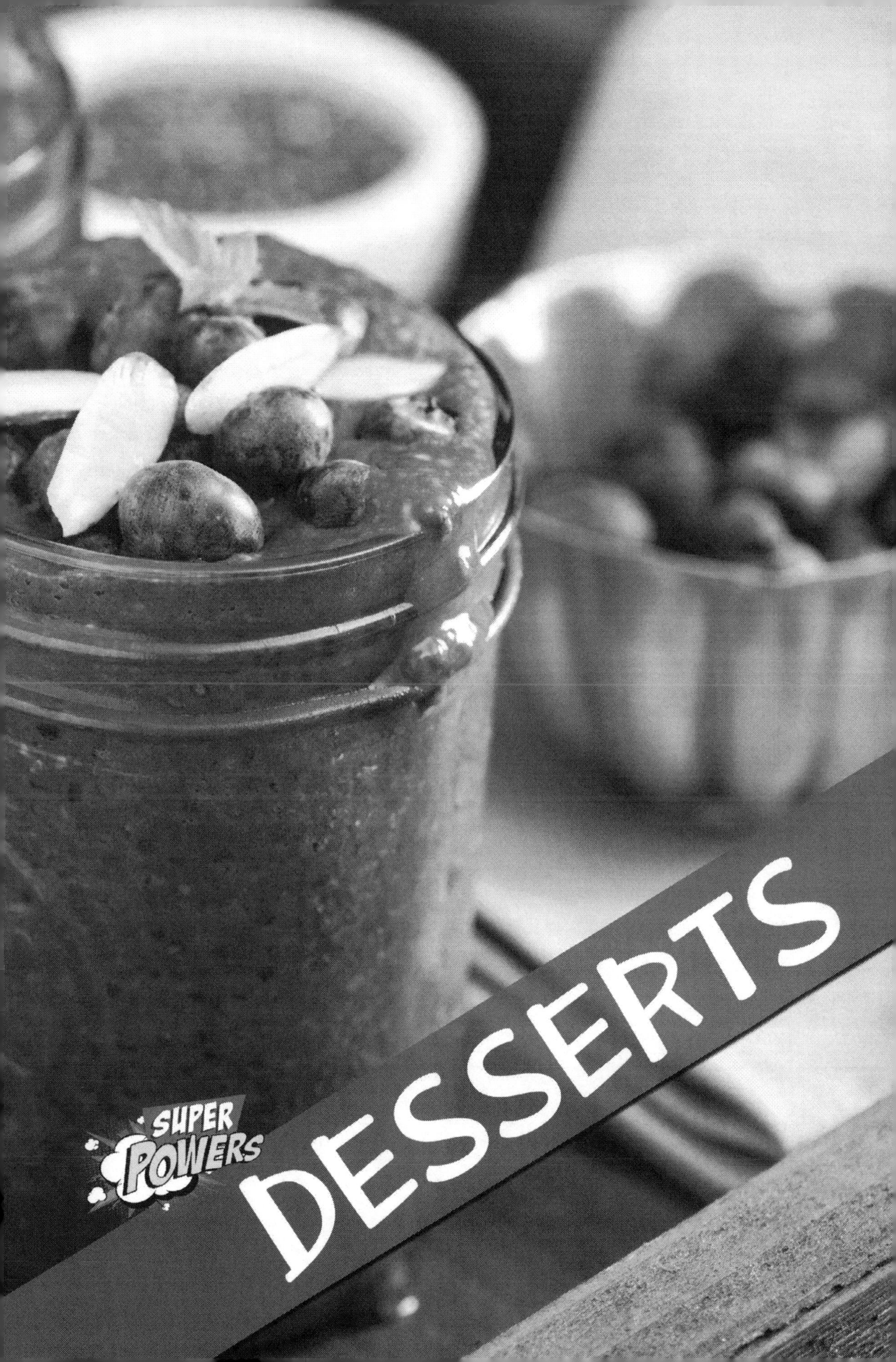

DESSERTS

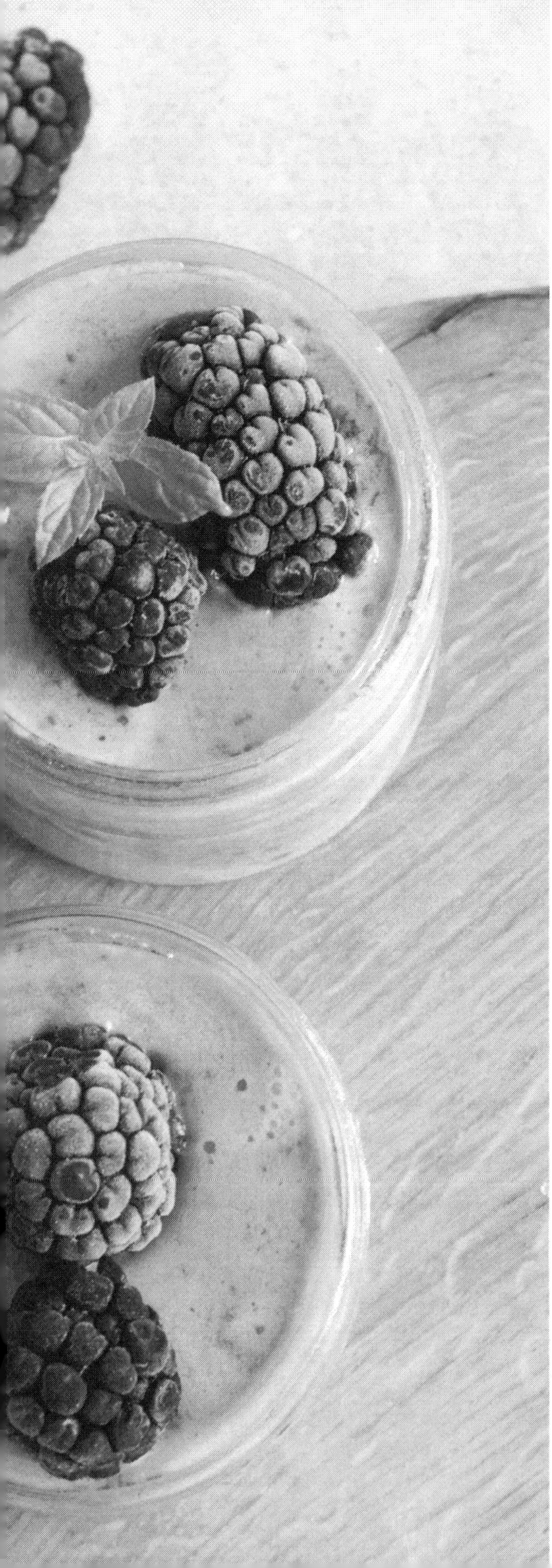

Sweet Cravings!

OK, one more thing we have not addressed that definitely deserves to be highlighted..... Sweet Cravings! Yes we all have them. Actually, there is a part of our brain that CRAVES sugar, or flour, or dairy when we are in the midst of total chaos! Yup, this is a common phenomenon and you, my friend, are not the only person in the entire world that this happens to. So I would like to give you some ammunition to keep this satisfied without the feeling like you are a typical "junkie".

First and foremost, your newly acquired consumption of high nutrient foods will help stabilize this... A little. Then your increase of protein and fat in each and every snack and meal will help keep this at bay... A little. So now let's top it off with some great treats that actually provide us with everything I have been preaching through all of these pages.

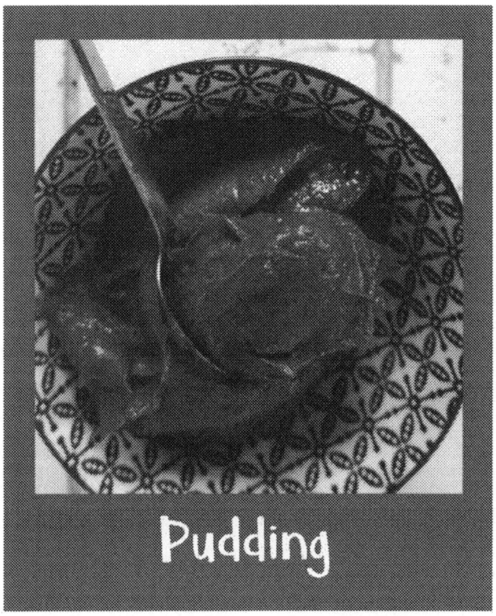

Chia Chocolate Pudding

Ingredients:

1 Cup Chia Seeds
1 1/2 Cup Coconut Milk
2 Tablespoons raw Cacao Powder
2 Tablespoons pureed Dates
1 Tablespoon Honey

Directions:

DF GF V

Mix all of the ingredients and place in the refrigerator to cool. The Chia seeds will end up absorbing all of the liquid. Once all of the liquid is absorbed, place the mixture into a high speed blender, and blend until smooth. You may need to add a bit of water or more coconut milk to improve the quality of the smoothness – do it gradually until desired smoothness is accomplished. *For a Protein Boost there are some amazing food based chocolate proteins you can add in (see resources in the back).

SUPERPOWER TIP: For extra sweetness puree some berries and mix it in with a swirl!

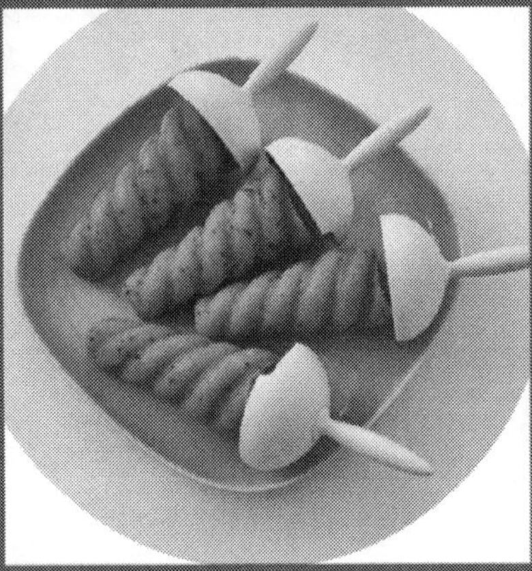

Frozen Fruit Pops

This is a Fun Filled Wild Card that you can easily enjoy and even share with a kid or two as long they are sweet enough, but the goal is to do this without added sugar and to include an adequate amount of protein.

Ingredients:

1. First let's start with the LIQUID – Coconut Water, Coconut Milk, Plain Water, Hemp Milk, or Almond Milk.

2. Here's what makes them SWEET – Dates, Pears, Bananas, Watermelon, Mango, and any other sweet fruit in season.

3. Here's what makes them POWERFUL – Goji Berries, Spinach, Kale, Collard Greens, Avocado, or Coconut.

4. Here's what gives it PROTEIN – Hemp Seeds, Raw Almond Butter, Raw Cashew Butter, plant based Protein Powder

Directions:

So this is what you do, for you first timers, start off by choosing a liquid that works for you and if you're in the mood to share with...the kids.

Next add in only fruit, make it tasty and blend it up in a high speed blender. Then add in a little bit of POWER and PROTIEN, blend it, taste it – if it's not sweet enough add in more fruit – Make it Tasty!

Then freeze it in Popsicle Sleeves or Ice Cube containers with toothpicks as handles. Now here's the trick, each time you make them add in more POWER and PROTIEN, your goal is to have an even mix of everything in a tasty treat that you love. My kids and I will eat several in a day and I love it – I know we are getting so much nutrition, that I couldn't be happier.

Now if you need a better, organized, plan then simply use one of the smoothie recipes on the previous pages and "Freeze them Up!!"

DF GF V NS

SUPERPOWER TIP: Use any of the Smoothie recipes that are listed in the Breakfast section or simply use your smoothie leftovers!

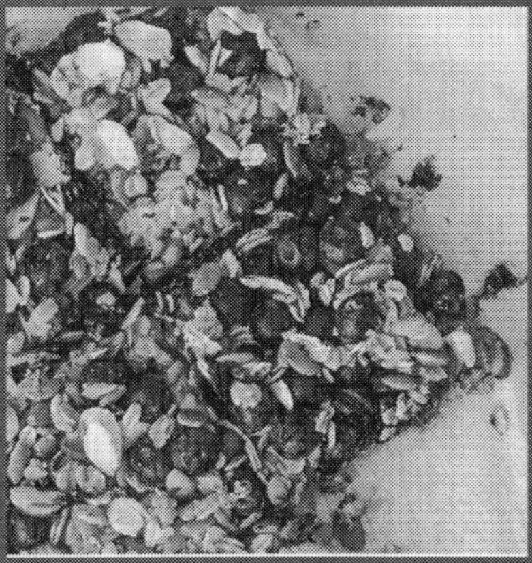

Snack Bars

Superfood Snack Bars – No Cooking Needed!

Ingredients:

1/2 Cup Dates (softened with a bit of water)
1/3 Cup freshly ground Flax Seeds
2 Tablespoons Coconut Butter
1/4 Cup Maple Syrup
1/2 Cup raw Almonds
1/2 Cup raw Pumpkin Seeds
1/4 Cup raw Chia Seeds
1/2 Cup organic raw Cacao Nibs
1/2 Cup organic Dried Blueberries
1/2 Cup Goji Berry
1/2 cup large flake unsweetened Dried Coconut
1/2 Cup Rolled Oats
1/4 to 1/2 Cup Water
*You can also add in a scoop of plant based protein powder for that extra punch of power!!

Directions:

First puree the dates in a high speed blender or food processor. Next add in the flax seeds, coconut butter, maple syrup and almonds. Mix everything well until you have a "pasty" type mixture. Then, stir in all of the remaining ingredients and add in just enough water to hold everything together.

Now there are a few ways you can set the mixture, you can spread on a dehydrator sheet about ½ inch thick and dehydrate for 10+ hours at 105 degrees or spread on a cookie sheet ½ inch thick and bake at 325 for 25 minutes (but this kills off the enzymes that you will have with the dehydrated version) or make one inch round balls, place on parchment papers, and refrigerate overnight.

DF GF V

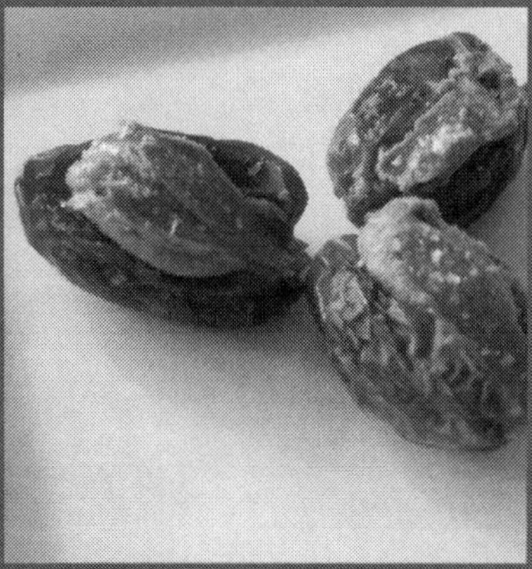

Dates

Dates Stuffed with Almond Butter

Talk about a simple treat, this one gets the prize. Take a few Medjool Dates, remove the pit and fill up with a teaspoon or so of Almond Butter. These stay fresh for a few weeks in an airtight container in the refrigerator.

DF GF V NS

Simple Sweet Treat

Ingredients:

1/3 Cup Honey
1/3 Cup Coconut Oil
1/2 Cup raw Cacao Powder
2 Tablespoons Chia Seeds
1/2 Cup raw Pumpkin Seeds
1/2 Cup raw Sunflower Seeds
1 Cup raw, Flaked Oats
1/2 Cup shredded unsweetened Coconut
1/2 Cup Dried Mulberries
Dash of Celtic Sea Salt

Directions:

First mix well the honey, coconut oil, and cacao powder with a spoon.

Next add in the remaining ingredients and mix those up as well.

And lastly you will make one inch balls, place them on parchment papers, and refrigerate overnight

DF GF V

SUPER POWERS

SHORT CUTS

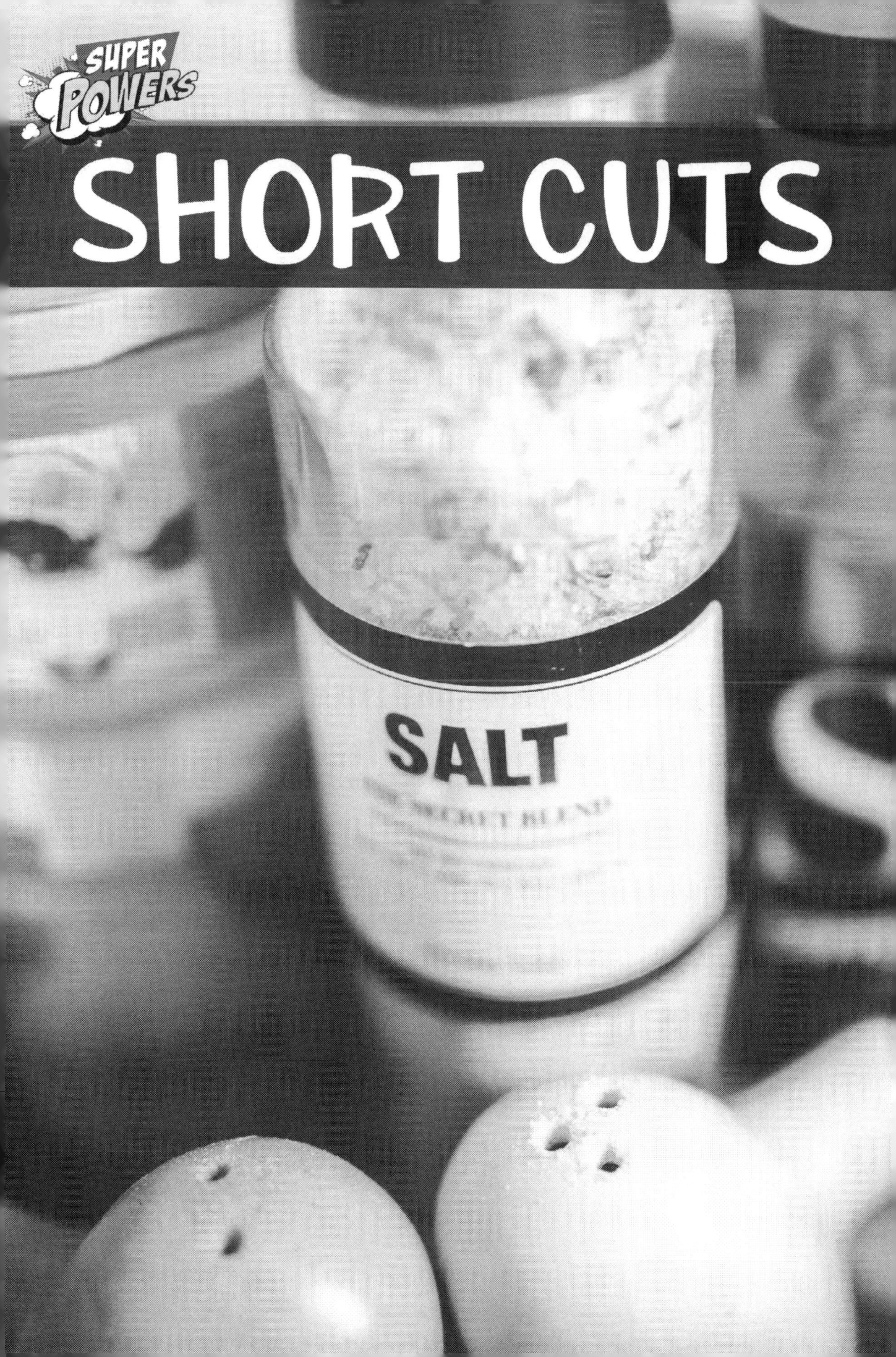

Think Outside of the SuperMarket

Supermarkets are no longer your only "go-to" location for fresh meats and produce. Here's a list of other amazing options to save you money, yet increase the quality of your foods

Co-ops – This is a cooperative business. They charge a membership fee, which gives you a SHARE of the bounty of fresh, organic produce and more. Your produce is typically available at a drop off point during a specific day of the week. This drop-off point could be a business down the street or your next door neighbor, each community is different

Butcher – A traditional meat market, a place where the butcher is king and they know their meats

Fish Market – Again, just like a meat market, a fish market specializes in fish and they know their product well

Health Food Store – These are more of a specialty and typically charge high rates

Online Retailer – Now here's where it can get good or bad. You have to do your homework, but once you find your vendors, you are set!

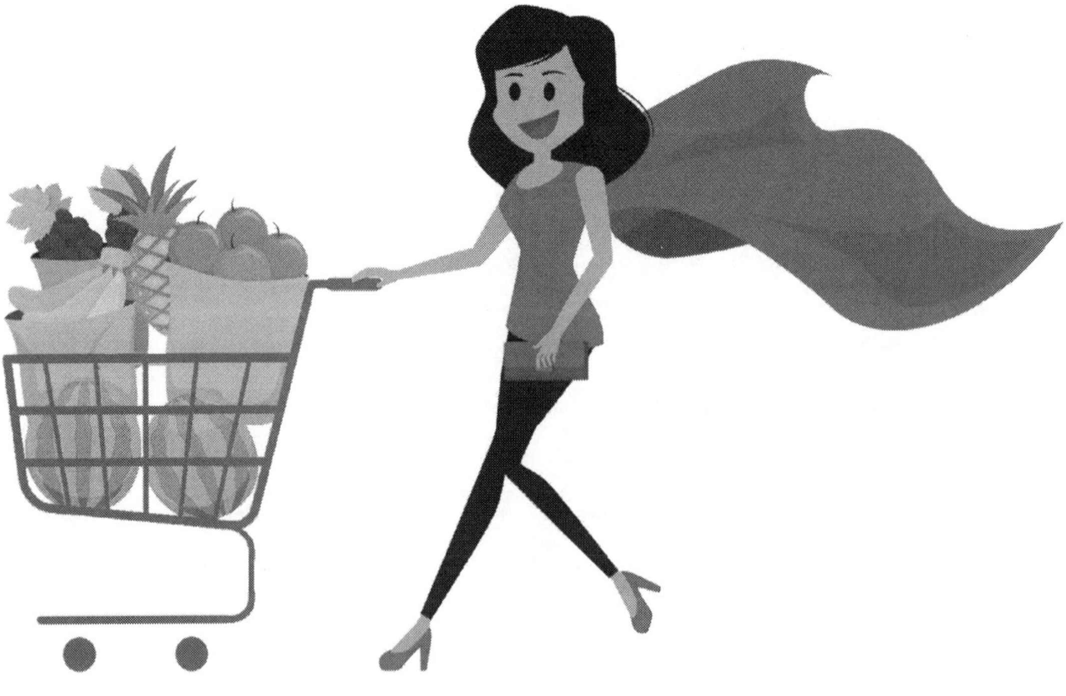

SUPER POWERS Pantry List

Your pantry is the Mecca of the kitchen, it is the basis of all recipes and all food plans. A well-stocked pantry will keep your food plan healthy and make sure that you have what you need for a well-designed meal, even when the pantry is at its emptiest!

The list below is designed simply as a guide, only you know what works best for you and your family. This list provides the basis of healthy cooking. Healthy cooking can be flavorful and easy. Be sure to choose organic when possible and read all ingredients lists—remember if you can't pronounce it and don't know what it is, don't eat it!

Basics

- Celtic or Himalayan Sea Salt – Fine and Coarse
- Black Peppercorns
- Extra Virgin Olive Oil – this one is for cooking
- Cold Pressed Olive Oil – this one is for salads or uncooked items
- Cold Pressed Coconut Oil – this one is for hundreds of things!
- Apple Cider Vinegar (with the mother – if you don't know what this is, don't worry the label will tell you)
- Red Wine Vinegar
- Balsamic or Sherry Vinegar
- Rice Vinegar (unseasoned)

Sweeteners

- Dates
- Coconut Sugar
- Maple Syrup
- Raw Honey
- Stevia Leaf – make the tea, store it and pour as your sweetener
- Organic Unsweetened Apple Sauce

Grains

- Basmati or Jasmin Rice
- Red or Black Rice
- Wild Rice
- Quinoa
- Organic Popcorn Kernels
- Organic Rolled Oats

Fruits and Nuts

- Dried Fruit: Mulberries, Golden Berries, Goji Berries
- Raw Seeds: Sunflower, Flax, Pumpkin, Chia, Sesame, or Hemp
- Raw Nuts – Almonds, Cashews, Walnuts, Pecans, Pine Nuts, Pistachios
- Raw Nut Butters - Almond, Cashew, Pecan

Packaged Goods

- Organic Chicken and Vegetable Broth
- Beans: Cannellini, Navy, Chickpeas or Black
- Lentils
- Olives or Capers
- Diced or Roasted Tomatoes
- Tomato Paste
- Tomato Sauce
- Sundried Tomatoes
- Roasted Red Peppers
- Spicy Mustard

Fresh or Dried Herbs and Spices

Keep in mind that fresh is always best, but the dried ones are great for backup. Dried Herbs are best kept for 1 yr.

- Bay leaves
- Cayenne Pepper
- Chili Powder
- Crushed Red Pepper
- Curry Powder
- Fennel or Dill Seed
- Granulated Garlic
- Ground Cinnamon
- Ground Cloves
- Ground Cumin
- Ground Ginger
- Ground Coriander
- Turmeric
- Vanilla Extract

- Oregano
- Basil
- Parsley
- Paprika
- Rosemary
- Thyme
- Whole Nutmeg

Fresh Produce

Should be seasonal, local, and organic, when possible. Here are some wonderful resources to find yours:

- http://www.epicurious.com/articlesguides/seasonalcooking/farmtotable/seasonalingredientmap
- http://www.micronutrients.com/wp-content/uploads/2015/07/ANDI-chart.pdf

But for the main staples of the home here are my top picks:

- Onions
- Garlic
- Avocados
- Carrots
- Celery
- Tomatoes
- Broccoli
- Bell Peppers
- Kale, Spinach, or Collard Greens
- Lettuce: Romaine, Boston or Mixed Greens
- Cilantro
- Gingerroot
- Potatoes: Sweet or Purple
- Lemons
- Apples
- Berries
- Bananas

Freezer

Remember that the freezer is a good place for backups and more. The following is a list of things that can be frozen without damaging the food.

- All Raw Nuts can be frozen to preserve shelf life
- If Fruit is getting a bit soft, remember to freeze it for smoothies – you can either puree the fruit and freeze in an ice tray then store in an air tight container or chop and store in an airtight container
- Rice, Grains, and any form of flour sometimes produce little bugs – by freezing these first you diminish the possibility of the bugs coming to life
- Frozen Peas, Broccoli and , Berries are always good backups to have

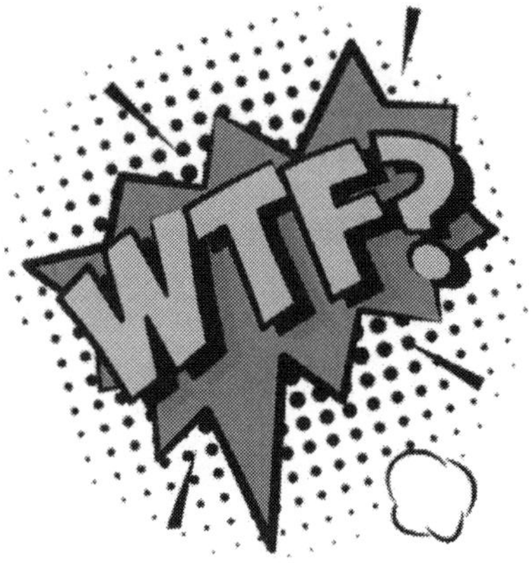

is in my Pantry?

Here's your NOT-SO-GOOD food list to live by:

- Expired food items
- Spices more than a year old
- Candy from 3 Halloweens ago, or even from a current purchase
- Twinkies, just in case
- Lard, the name says it all
- Anything with corn syrup or high fructose corn syrup
- Minute Rice - Quick Oats - Roasted Nuts or Seeds
- Any canned goods with more than 500mg of salt
- Any seasoning or packaged food item with MSG - Monosodium glutamate
- Packaged foods with food colorings
- Packaged foods with words you cannot pronounce and have no idea what the H%*@ they mean
- Creamer or half and half
- Traditional Mayo or Ketchup

SUPER POWERS Substitution List

For every "not so healthy" thing we can choose, we can easily choose something that will give us the same satisfaction while ramping up our SuperPowers. So here it is; these are my favorite swaps to make eating a pleasure!

Avocado mash *for mayo*

Mayonnaise has about 200 plus calories, while the same serving of avocado only brings in about half of that with an array of essential vitamins and minerals ... hmmm. So without giving it a thought, smash up an avocado and add it anyplace you would use mayo!

Arugula, romaine, spinach, collards and kale *for iceberg lettuce*

Darker green leaves are packed full of nutrients like iron, vitamin C, and antioxidants. The pale leaves of iceberg lettuce have no chance to even compare. Make each bite count and go for the nutrient dense varieties!

Coconut milk *for cream*

Coconut milk is a great exchange for heavy cream in soups and stews. It may bring a bit of coconut flavor but not so much that you can't cover up with spices and more.

Lettuce leaves *for tortilla wraps*

Any wrap dish or taco can be replaced with a large lettuce or greens leaf! Here's a great way to lower the processed carbs and enhance the nutrition.

Nuts *for croutons (in salads)*

Have you seen my famous nut mix? Yup, it's an ideal way of adding protein and quality fat to a salad without the carbs and additives that croutons bring. Take an array of raw nuts and seeds and blend them into a coarse powder and have at it! Check out my video at http://youtu.be/9W9IGbd2qp0

Pureed fruit *for syrup*

Syrup for pancakes and syrup for waffles ... who needs syrup when you can take some fresh berries and puree them up for a sweet delight?

Quinoa *for oatmeal*

You can easily cook quinoa with water or any nut milk then add it into mashed up berries and you have a great protein filled breakfast.

Quinoa *for couscous*

Couscous is made from processed wheat flour; quinoa is a whole-grain superfood packed with protein and nutrients. They have the same texture but quinoa gives you so much more nutrition per bite!

Rolled oats *for breadcrumbs*

As I always say, minimize the gluten! Traditional breadcrumbs are filled with all sorts of additives and more; on the other hand, rolled oats can be seasoned up with herbs to make an amazing breading alternative.

Spaghetti squash *for pasta*

Roasted and pulled apart with a fork, spaghetti squash is a great low-carb and lower-calorie substitute for pasta. One squash will make between two and three servings.

Ideas for Snack Items

Frozen grapes *for a summertime snack*

Freeze grapes without the stems and pass out the bags for a great snack on a hot day. Who needs candy?

Frozen smoothie *for frozen ice pops*

As long as they are sweet your kids will love them, so take full advantage. Add in greens like collard green or cilantro, and then sweeten with dates and bananas and add in other fruits in between. I even add in protein powder for that extra bonus.

Kale chips *for potato chips*

Once you have gone kale, there is no turning back! Toss in olive oil with seasonings of your choice, place on a flat pan or cookie sheet, then broil on low—but keep your eye on the prize, they only take a few minutes and can burn very easily. This will become your "go-to" crunch snack with less fat than any potato chip out there!

Ideas for Baking

Almond flour / Nut flour *for wheat flour*

Too much gluten is not a good thing so here is a great way to up the protein and omega-3s in most of your baked goods! Keep in mind that the flavor is a bit nuttier than traditional flour and almond flour is much heavier, so when making your exchange think about using a 1/4 cup at the beginning (so 1 cup flour would become 3/4 cup flour and 1/4 cup almond flour). Or, if you want to take it full force and your recipe includes a rising agent, you may need to increase the amount of rising agent (by about 1/2 teaspoon per cup of almond flour added) to account for the extra weight. (**Nut flours do tend to be heavier than traditional flour, so make sure to up the amount of baking powder and baking soda in the recipe so the dough can rise as normal)

Avocado puree *for butter (in anything chocolate!)*

This is best done on any type of fudge or chocolate recipe so that the flavor of the avocado does not shine through. This exchange may take a few trial runs to get it right, but for the most part a 1:1 ratio works well.

Black beans *for flour in brownies!*

Ditch the flour and add a can of black beans instead (drained and rinsed) in your favorite brownie recipe. This makes for a great way to pack in the protein and give a good kick to the gluten. When baking, exchange 1 cup of flour for 1 cup or a 15oz can of organic black beans and puree.

Cacao nibs *for chocolate chips*

The root of chocolate started out as cacao nibs. This unprocessed alternative cuts out all of the additives, fat, and other stuff and leaves you with a nutrient dense alternative. You have to play around with this one and make sure to sweeten it, but the sky's the limit as to what things you can make!

Chia seeds *for eggs*

It's more than your traditional Chia Pet. Combine 1 tablespoon chia seeds with 1 cup of water and let sit for 15 minutes to create a perfect 1:1 egg substitute for baking.

Coconut flour *for flour*

If you're looking at enhancing nutrients and removing some of the carbs from a baked treat, coconut flour works well as a partial exchange. Be careful though—using more than 1/2 a cup at a time could allow the flour's bitterness to take over. Your exchange can be tricky so be sure to add an equal amount of extra liquid! For baking, you typically want to substitute only 1/4 to 1/3 cup of coconut flour for your 1 cup of traditional flour (so if it's ¼ cup coconut flour, then you also have an additional ¾ cup of your traditional flour).

Dates *for sugar*

It takes about 10 dates to exchange one cup of sugar but this also gives you a bit of protein, tons of fiber, vitamins A, B, and K, folate, magnesium, phosphorus, potassium, and a lot more! So for the added nutrients and fiber this is a perfect exchange, the calories are about the same but the benefits are so much more!

Flax meal *for eggs*

Here's a vegan trick, mix 1 tablespoon of freshly ground flax seeds with 3 tablespoons of warm water and whisk well to combine. Next, let it sit in the refrigerator for 5-10 minutes before using as an exchange for 1 egg in any baked recipe.

Mashed bananas *for fats*

With a 1:1 ratio a perfectly soft and ripe banana can help the same way as avocados to replace the fat in a baking recipe. The consistency works well and the nutritional punch adds in potassium, fiber, and vitamin B6.

Meringue *for frosting*

Typical frosting can add in a good 300 plus calories to a basic cup cake, ugh! Meringue is made from egg whites and sugar; it's a great fat-free substitution for traditional frosting. Want to make it even cooler? Light a torch to it and that bit of charred delight will bring out the sweetness and caramelized flavor.

Unsweetened applesauce *for baking*

- Using applesauce instead of sugar can give you all the sweetness with none of the added sugar, and that means fewer calories as well! One cup of applesauce contains only about 100 calories; a cup of sugar, on the other hand, can add in more than 700 calories! This exchange is ideal for cookies, muffins and more. The exchange is a 1:1 ratio, but for every cup of applesauce, cut down on the amount of liquid in the recipe by 1/4 cup or so.

- Want to eliminate the fat? Try applesauce instead of butter or oil in recipes like sweet bread, muffins, and more. Don't jump in full force at first, try exchanging only half the fat the first time around and see how that goes (so if you need 1 cup butter, try ½ cup applesauce and ½ cup butter). On the next round you'll know just how much works for your recipe.

Vanilla *for sugar*

Considering one cup of sugar can be about 800 calories, now think about cutting that in half and replacing it with vanilla extract. Now, it's a challenging exchange and may take a few trials on your part, but you can start by cutting 2 tablespoons of sugar and adding an extra 1/2 teaspoon of vanilla extract.

Your SuperPower Food Plan

Now that we have some form of a foundation for your food plan, this is a sample of what mine looks like. Don't get fixated on what I do; the most important part of all of this is for you to create the right plan that works for you, your life, and your triumphs! Some of you may need more variety; some of you may need more meat, play with it. The key is that your food should help you:

- Stabilize Your Energy
- Keep Your Energy Constant Throughout the Day
- Remove some of the Moodiness (granted sometimes it's well deserved, but not every day, all day!)
- Maintain a Feeling of Clear-Headedness
- Keep Your Immune System Strong and Powerful
- And, of course, my favorite, SuperPower the Ability to Conquer ALL in a Single Bound!

DAY	MONDAY	TUESDAY	WEDNESDAY
First AM	2 Glasses of Water	2 Glasses of Water	2 Glasses of Water
Breakfast	2 Soft Boiled Eggs and A Protein Smoothie	Muesli with Hemp Milk and 1 Hardboiled Egg	2 Sunny Side Up Eggs and a Green Smoothie
Mid-Morning Snack	Apple with Almond Butter	Trail Mix	Banana with Raw Walnut Butter
Mid-Day Meal	Part 2 of Morning Smoothie	Salad with Romaine, Avocado, Tomatoes, Olive Oil, and Nut Mix	Part 2 of Morning Smoothie
Afternoon Snack	Walnuts	Hummus and Celery	Roasted Seaweed with Avocado
Evening Meal	Beans and Rice with fresh Kale and tomatoes	Roasted Brussel Sprouts with White Beans and Sundried Tomatoes	Baked Salmon with Broccolini
Liquids	6 Glasses of Water, 2 Cups of Tea, 1 Coconut Water, 1 Kombucha	6 Glasses of Water, 2 Cups of Tea, 1 Coconut Water, 1 Kombucha	6 Glasses of Water, 2 Cups of Tea, 1 Coconut Water, 1 Kombucha

TAKE NOTE: My food plan works for me, my activity level, and the time between meals

THURSDAY	FRIDAY	SATURDAY	SUNDAY
2 Glasses of Water	2 Glasses of Water	2 Glasses of Water	2 Glasses of Water
Omelet with Tomatoes and Asparagus	2 Soft Boiled Eggs and A Protein Smoothie	2 Sunny Side Up Eggs with Sautéed Onions and Tomatoes	Oats with berries and Nut Mix
Cashews and Mulberries	Infinity Greens Bar	Apple with Almond Butter	Smoothie from Yesterday
Quinoa with Mixed Greens and Tomatoes	Salad with Romaine, Avocado, Tomatoes, Olive Oil, and Nut Mix	Green Smoothie	Vegetable Sushi Roll with 3 Pieces of Salmon Sushi
Almond Butter and Dates	Vegetable Sushi Roll	Trail Mix	Chopped Mango and Walnuts
Salad with Romaine, Avocado, Tomatoes, Shrimp, Olive Oil, and Nut Mix	Stuffed Squash with White Beans and Veggies	Quinoa with Sautéed Vegetables	Roasted Chicken and Veggies
6 Glasses of Water, 2 Cups of Tea, 1 Coconut Water, 1 Kombucha	6 Glasses of Water, 2 Cups of Tea, 1 Coconut Water, 1 Kombucha	6 Glasses of Water, 2 Cups of Tea, 1 Coconut Water, 1 Kombucha	6 Glasses of Water, 2 Cups of Tea, 1 Coconut Water, 1 Kombucha

Thoughts to Ponder

As you formulate your plan, think of the following:

- If there is a large amount of time between meals or you know you will be going non-stop, then add in more fat and protein to that initial meal. You never want to get to your next meal feeling famished; if you do then you'll know you needed to alter the proportions of carbohydrates, proteins, and quality fats in the meal before.

- If you are sick or have been sick due to a disease or illness add in more protein for repair.

- If you have a big workout planned and want the energy to JAM, add in more carbs from fruits or veggies with your protein and fats.

- If there will be a small amount of time between meals, make that meal higher in carbs from fruit and vegetables because they will break down and metabolize quickly and leave you ready for the next dish!

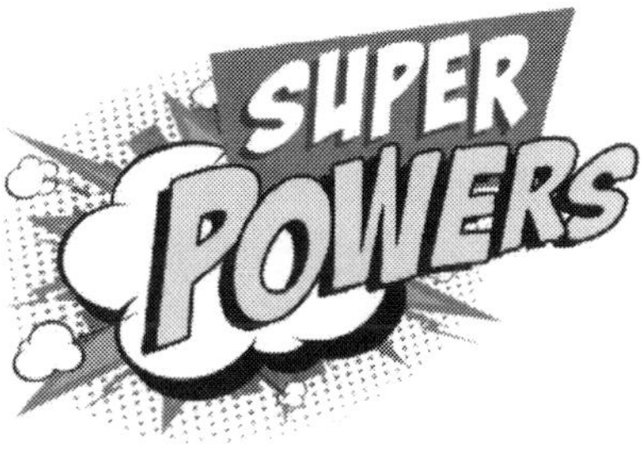

Kitchen Quick Fix List

In order to easily make smooth transitions in the kitchen, which can be tough at times, and avoiding all the TV commercials that sell you the easiest foods to buy and die from, I have my list of a few of my favorite tricks to keep the family dinners on time and yummy without keeping yourself stuck in the kitchen for hours to come.

Cook enough plain quinoa for a least two meals – Quinoa will stay fresh and ready to go in the refrigerator for up to 5 days as long as you cooked it and stored it plain.

Chopped onions and garlic will last in an airtight container for about a week and they can last even longer in the freezer.

Cooked rice (although this should never be a main staple of a meal, just a side accessory) can also be cooked plain and stored for about 5 days in the fridge.

Roasted potatoes (or roasted sweet potatoes, even better) can be kept in the fridge for about 4 days, then, when you want to use them again, sauté with a splash of water to bring them back to life.

Hardboiled eggs with the shells intact can last in the fridge for 5 days.

Review my storage techniques for veggies a few pages back, for your quick salad and sautéed veggie alternatives.

Cooking a whole chicken can leave you with leftovers for a salad, wrap or a quick snack. And for those weeks that seem never to end, just buy an organic roasted chicken, already done, super easy.

When you sauté vegetables make a bit extra – granted, it will only last in the fridge for a couple of days but it rocks for a wrap or salad on the go

Work on some "batch cooking" favorites – that's cooking extra, for those who haven't heard of this before. Then freeze each serving so that you can easily thaw out a serving and serve it up!

Hunger 101

OK and one last thing, it's a biggie, something we may overlook... How HUNGRY are you? Yup, I asked it, and I did that because many times hunger is stress, anxiety or something else in drag. We can easily be truly hungry but we can, just as easily, be hungry for a totally different reason. Hunger appears for one of the following reasons:

- Real Hunger
- Dehydration
- Vitamin Deficiency
- Comfort
- Stress and Anxiety
- Or simply from feeling overwhelmed!

And there you have it, as crazy as this seems, many of us lead these hectic lives and need to make do the best we can. Some of you may be blessed with more time, but my crew of SuperWomen takes charge, moves forward, and conquers the world, so we need every second that is available and more. Food should be one of the things that fuels us; instead of overindulging or running from it, it is there to make you the best YOU that you can be. So rather than eating for comfort and sanity, eat to build strength, emanate power, and show off those SuperWoman traits that make you OUTSTANDING! With every single meal and snack you, my friend, want to eat to feel satisfied NOT FULL! Got it?

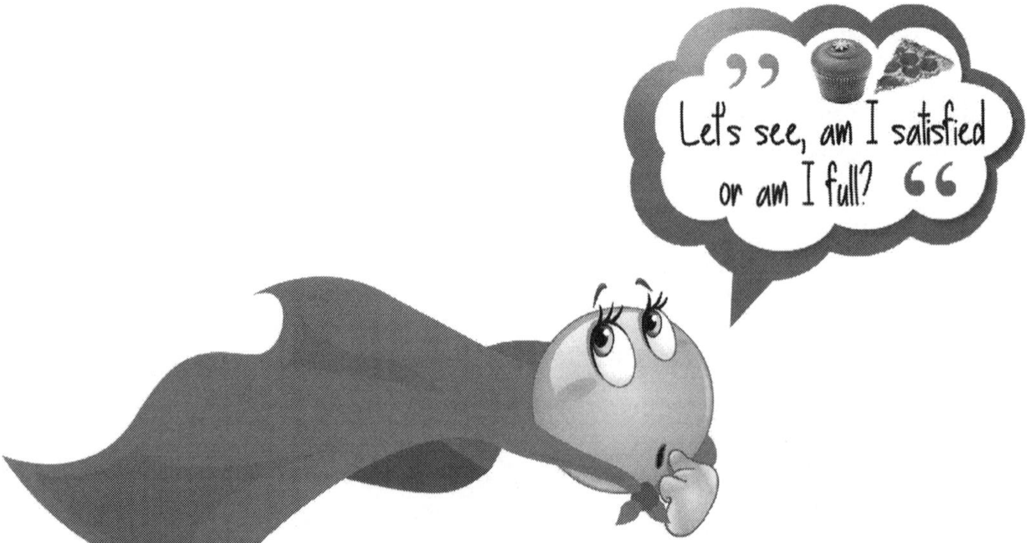

SuperPowers Recap

Flour, sugar, dairy, and alcohol all break down as a sugar and too much sugar WILL make you fat, slow, and lacking in your SuperPowers, for sure.

Set yourself up for success, all meals and snacks should have a balanced amount of carbohydrates from fruits and vegetables, proteins, and a small amount of quality fats to sustain your energy centers.

If you're eating late at night and heading straight for bed, keep your meal light, easy to digest, something like a salad that won't sit in your stomach while you sleep. Remember, if it sits there without a purpose, your body will simply store it as fat.

NO JUNK AT HOME! Keep your pantry as a healthy oasis of wonderful, energizing SuperPower choices.

Meal prep, meal prep, meal prep – It is all about setting yourself up with a system and then making it a set task for the week to ramp up your energy centers. Avoid looking at this like a chore, it is a way for you to energize your body and keep your mind as sharp as a whip!

If you're like me, you're always on the go; make it a plan to pack your food or at least a decent snack to hold you over until you get home.

"The Body is designed

to move with ease,

to live with enthusiasm,

and to play at any age"

-Adita Lang ♡

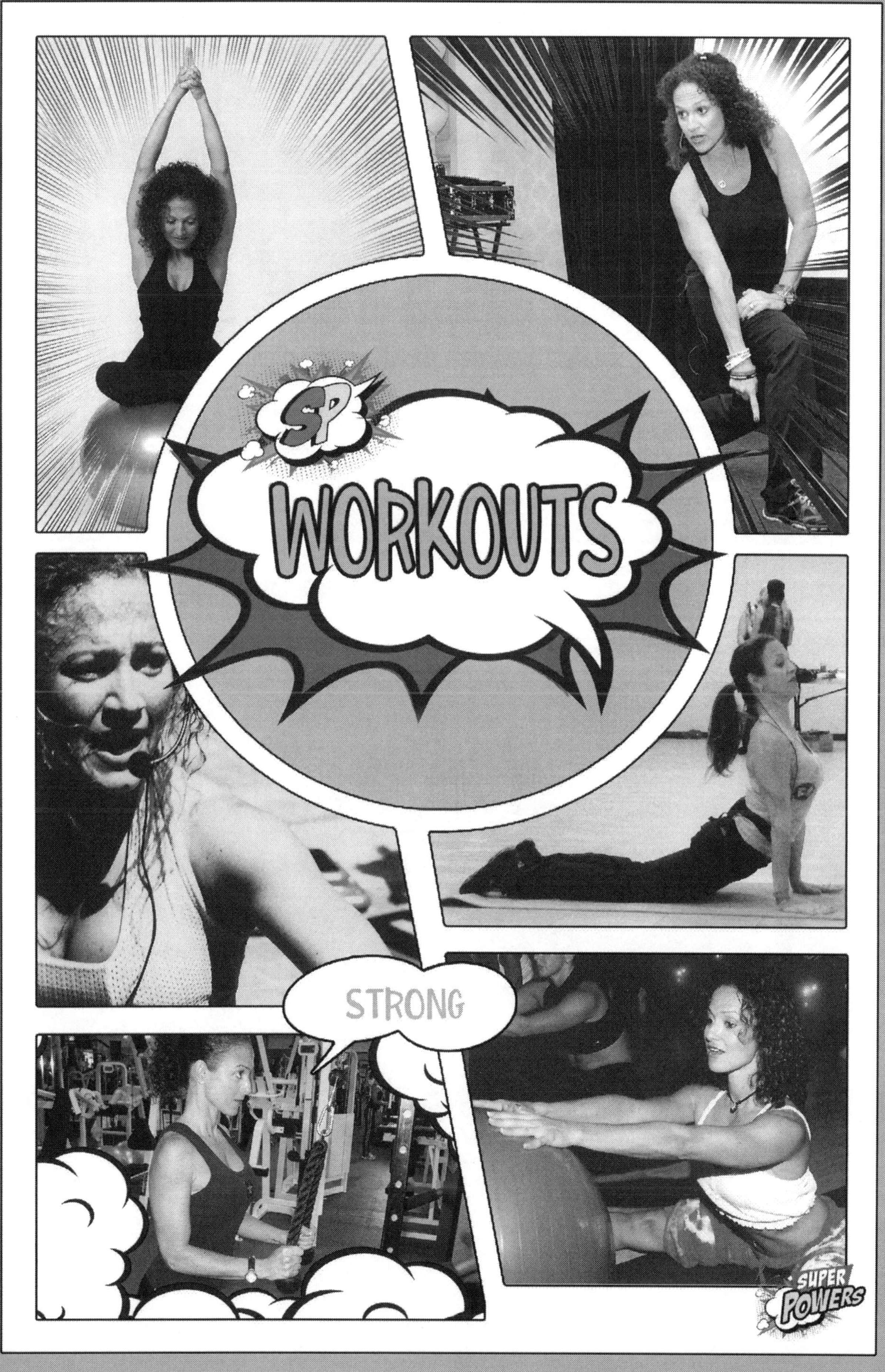
SP
WORKOUTS
STRONG
SUPER POWERS

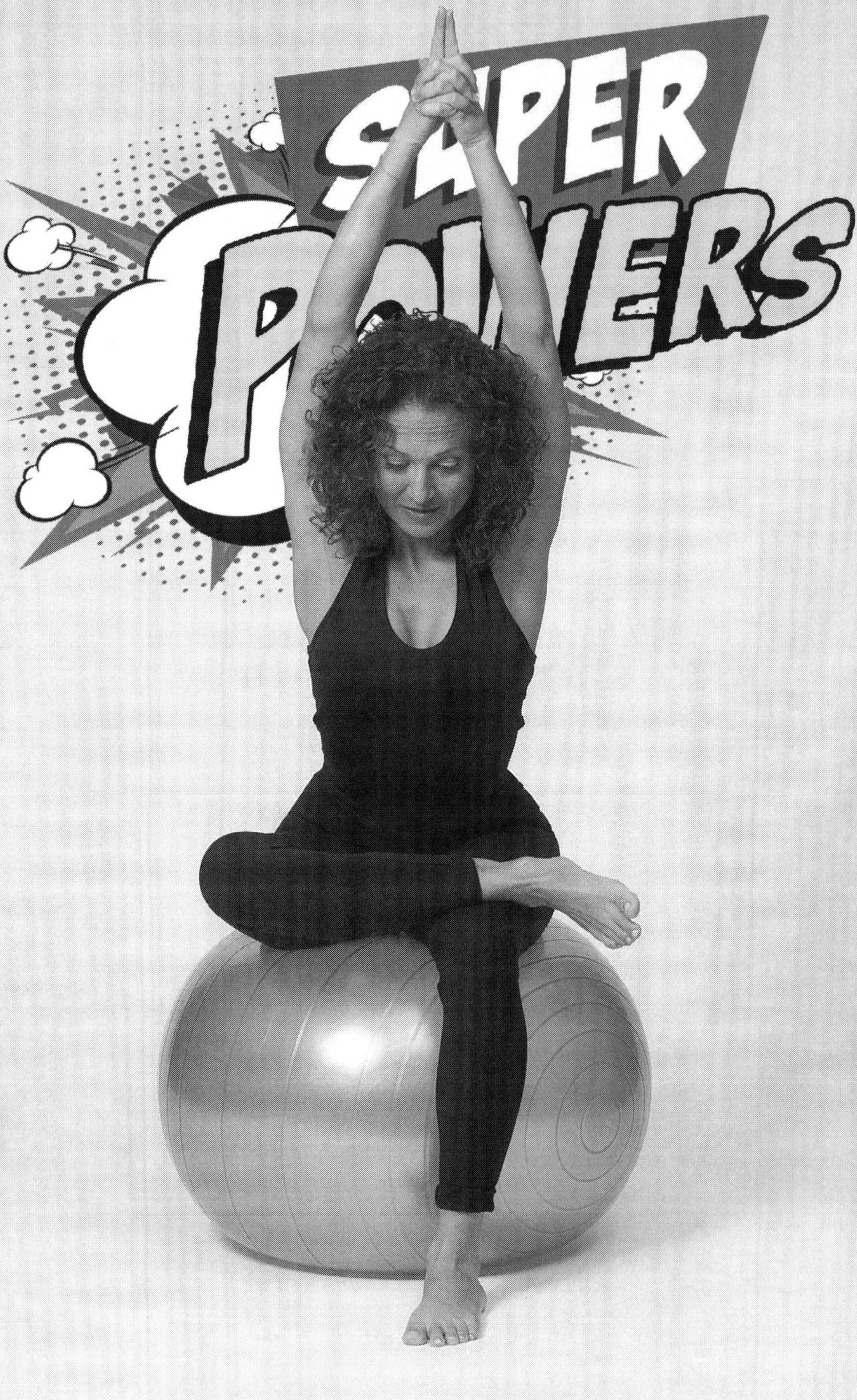

SuperPower Workouts

Ugh, I know that for some this may seem tedious and for others it's the highlight of their day, but either way our bodies are designed to move. Fluidity of movement is that thing that gives us strength in the muscles and encourages elimination of toxins and fat. Think of exercise as your "happy pill"; the endorphins that you get from each and every exercise session help you kick off the stress and charge forward with clarity.

During my pregnancies I had to give up the intensity in my training regime and sometimes bring it to a complete halt. Now jump forward a few years and add in two kids and time became my enemy. I wanted my old life of training back, 20 hours a week that I had drenched my body with sweat and loved every minute of it. But there was a new reality, time was at a minimum, yet my body craved fluid movement. I had no choice but to release myself from expectations and simply fit in what I could, when I could, and be happy with it. I spent years with an unbalanced approach to health; it was now time to create a plan that worked with my day to day and start anew.

What Makes a Good Exercise Program? A good exercise program should be comprised of cardiovascular/endurance type exercise, strength training, and flexibility. Your cardiovascular conditioning encourages circulation, strength adds power to that circulation, and flexibility opens the body to receive all of the benefits of that circulation. There are hundreds of programs out there, it is just a matter of a bit of trial and error and finding just the right one to inspire you and keep you going. But here's the thing, traditional exercise programs in a gym are not your only solution or option; your goal is to sweat, increase your heart rate, and lift heavy things. Hmmm, that's right; a good gardening session could work wonders, not to mention housecleaning, home repairs, throwing kids around, and more. A good combination of structured exercise and other things can provide a well-rounded program for most people! The old standby of performing 60 minutes of consecutive exercise has now changed to a "friendlier" approach; small bouts of exercise throughout the day are just as good. So if 10 minutes is all you have at the moment—that works. The American College of Sports Medicine promotes 150 minutes of exercise per week for the novice enthusiast, how you break it down is up to you.

A SuperWoman's Muscle Building Plan for Triumph

The ones that help you run in 10 directions while jumping over the hurdles of your day and still leaving you looking fiercer than ever!

For every pound of muscle you have on your frame, you burn 50 calories doing nothing. The goal is to make your body as efficient as possible; as I mentioned earlier, you want your metabolism to turn on as much as you can. The two things that will rev it up are food and exercise! You can easily do a set of squats while brushing your teeth; I'll bet money that you have done some other weird things during that time before. I think if you let go of the old drudgery of "this is the only way to exercise" and move more towards "this is the best way for me to incorporate exercise" you'll come to love the benefits and not feel the pressure of it all. The bottom line is you just need to move with a little bit more force than your traditional stroll in the park, and voila... Calories burned, heart rate up, and muscles stronger. If you have the time you can easily do a full 60 minutes of activity, but if that doesn't match your needs then breaking it down to small bouts of exercise and movement throughout the day will do the trick. Once you rev up that metabolism you can sit back and listen to your engines purr.

True SuperWomen Techniques for Success

To maximize every benefit possible with movements, exercise, and lifting anything heavy there are just a few things I would like you to understand:

1. **Technique is everything.** This is what will make you strong, but this is also what will keep you injury free. Your basic technique for all movement is this:

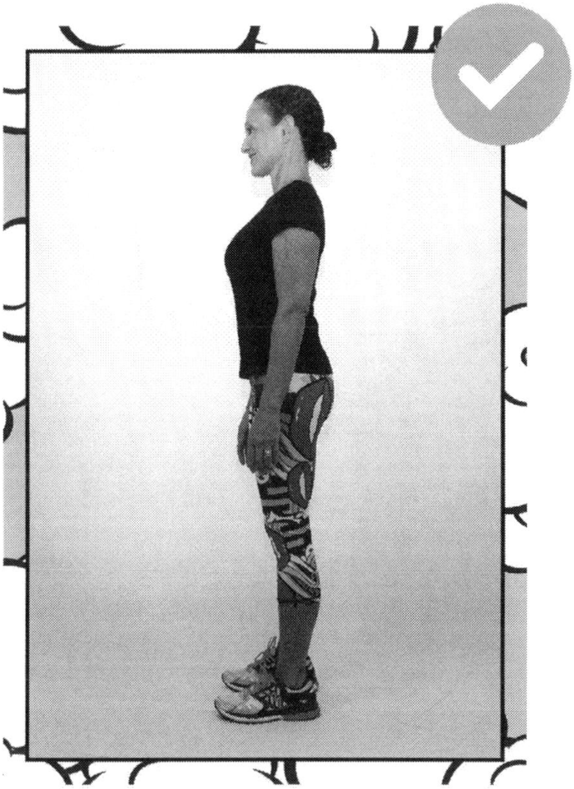

Posture

- Shoulders back and down away from your ears.
- Chest is lifted and proud, no matter what size it is.
- Abdominals are held in tight by contracting the rib cage and the belly button together.
- And your pubic bone should be aiming away from you, either straight down to the floor from a standing position or parallel to the floor from a lying down position.

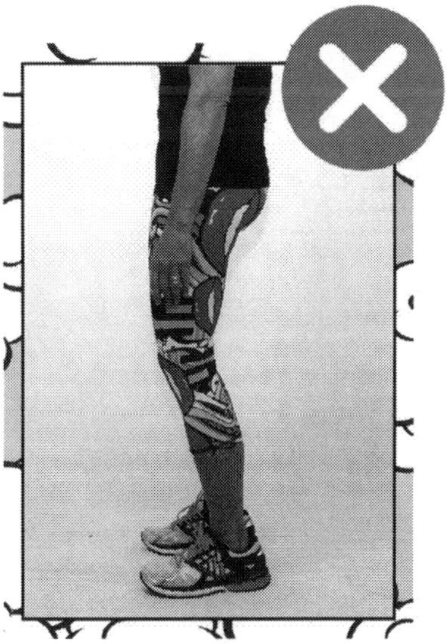

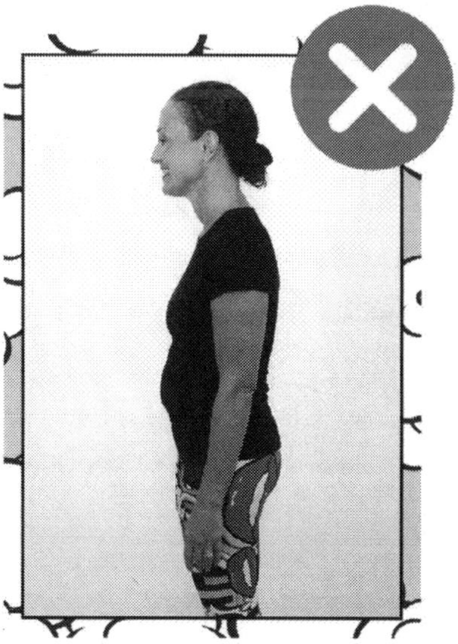

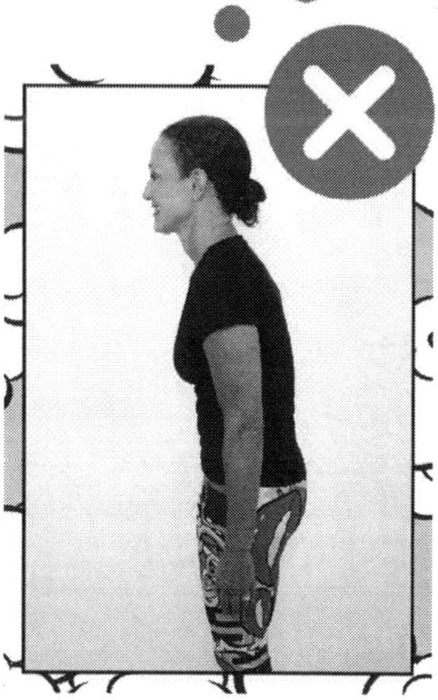

- In addition your head is centered with your ears over your shoulders and if you're standing the weight of your body is evenly distributed throughout your feet.

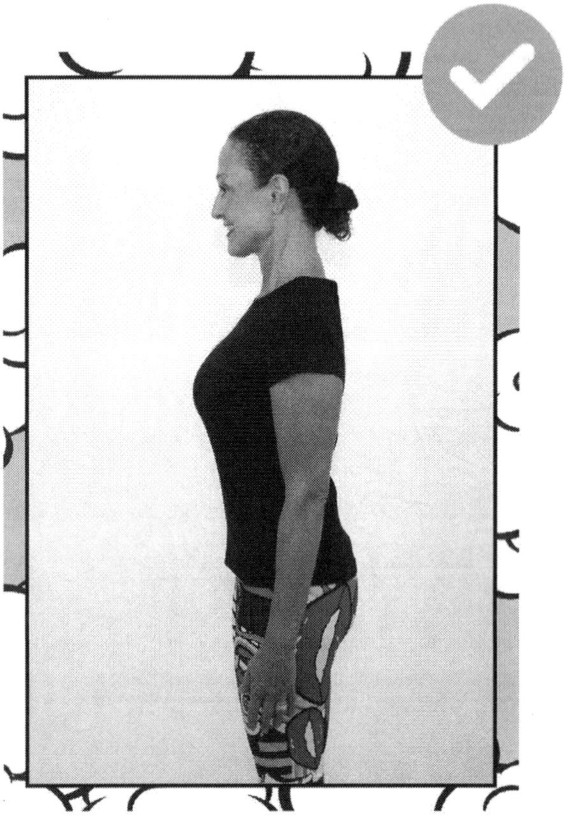

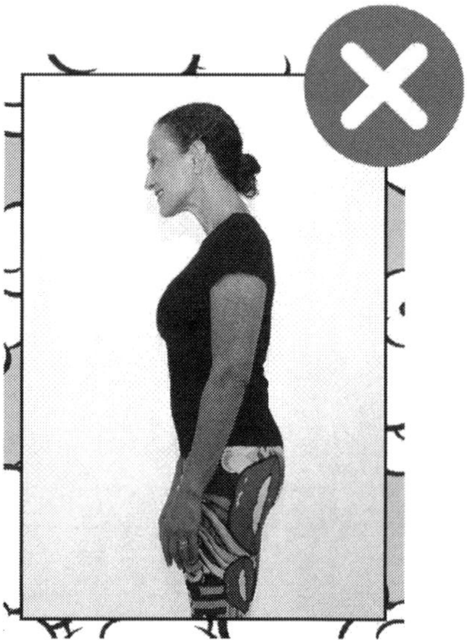

2. **Now, when performing any form of repetition, don't rush through it.** This is the one time that s-l-o-w-i-n-g down actually produces the best benefits. Movements should be slow, controlled, and perfectly executed!

3. **Use your breathing to dictate the speed of your movement.** Try to breathe with your movements, inhale with one part and exhale with the other. This will help you slow down your repetitions and teach you to bring in enough oxygen to burn the fat and enhance the muscle!

SUPER POWERS Exercises

Here are my top 10 SUPERPOWER moves that require no equipment:

Squat This is basically what you do when you sit down in a chair or on a toilet; the only difference is that you don't get that chance to slouch into it and relax. The minute that tush touches down it's time to get back up and do it again.

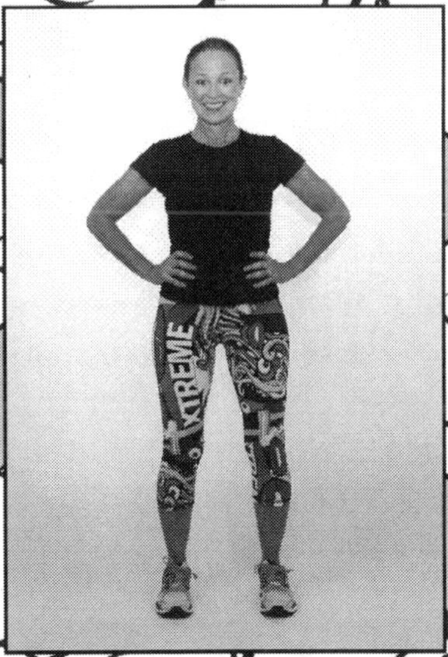

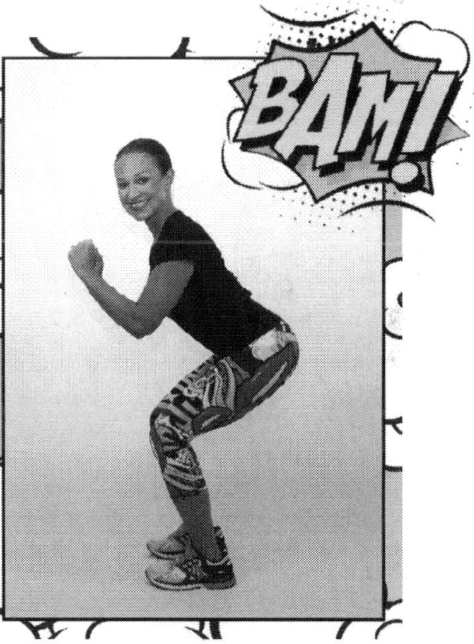

Lunges No droopy booty here! Get that tush perky and round. From a standing position with your feet hip width apart, step one foot forward, bending both knees and keeping the back knee just a few inches from the floor; step it back and do the other leg.

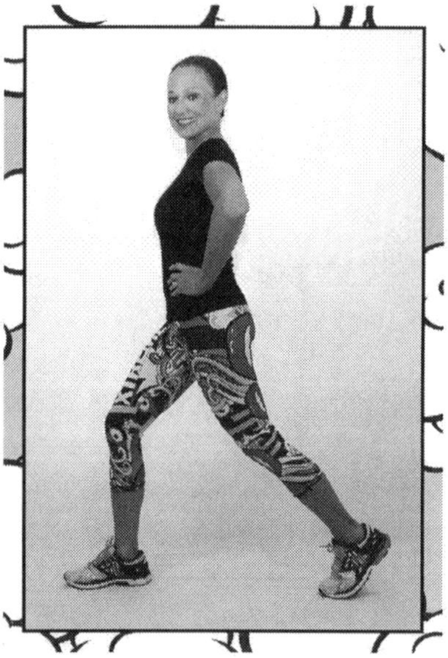

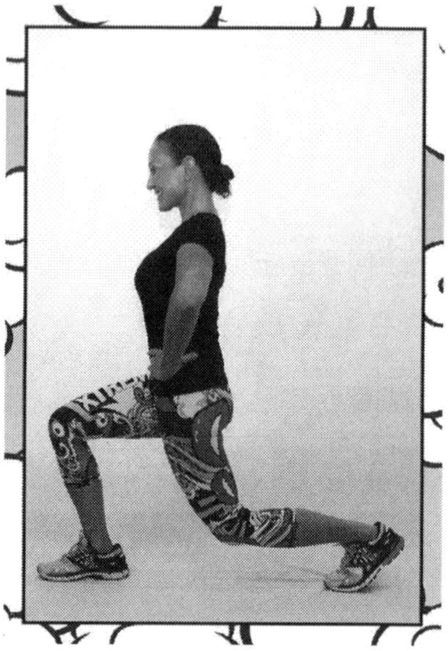

Plie + Inner Thighs I love this one. From a standing position, open your legs so wide that when you bend your knees you have two 90 degree bends in the knees. As you begin to straighten the legs focus on contracting the tush; then, when you bend again, think about opening your knees wider. You will do about 10 or so then stay with both knees bent and slightly push the knees in and out for another 10 reps or so.

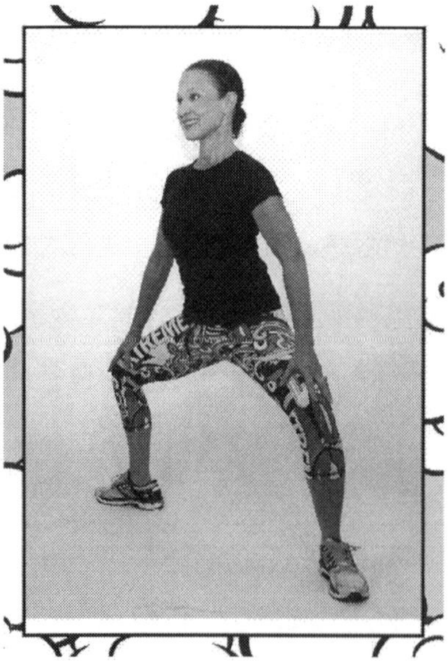

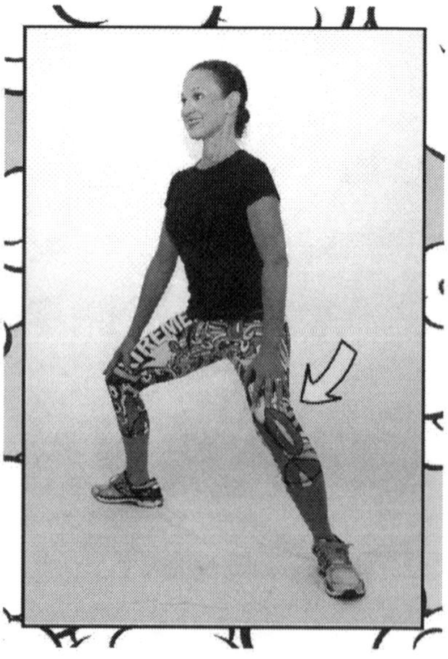

Single Leg Extension From a standing position, balance your weight on one leg and hold the opposing knee up. Take that knee and begin to straighten the leg, focusing on tightening up the muscles at the top of your thighs. Bend again and repeat for about 10 reps then move on to the other leg.

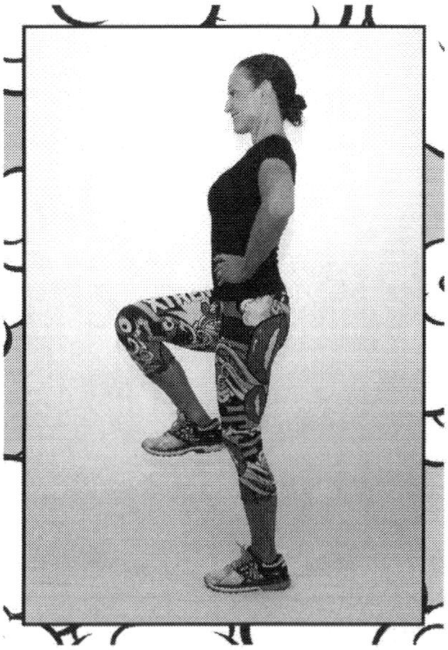

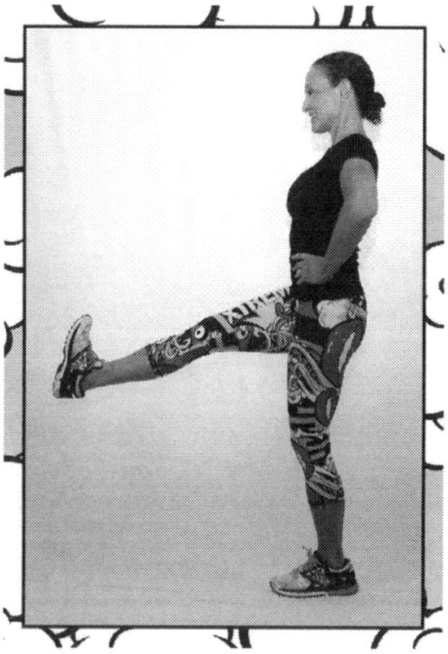

Single Leg Rotation Start from the same position as the leg extension above. Instead of extending the leg, this time try to rotate the hip so that the foot moves in front of the stabilizing leg. Do about 10 rotations on each leg.

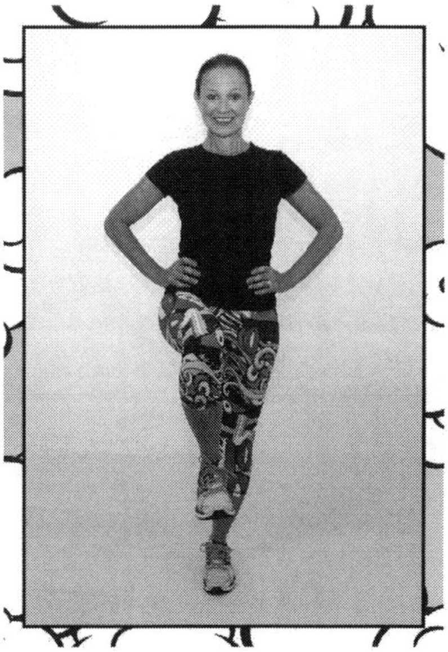

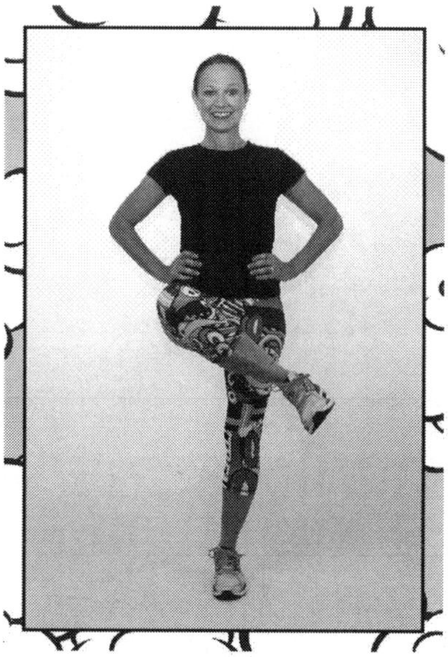

Push Ups The ultimate vanity part fixer upper. You can do them from your knees or your toes; your torso is in a straight line with your thighs and your hands are open wide enough so that when you bend your elbow, you have a clean 90 degree bend.

Modified

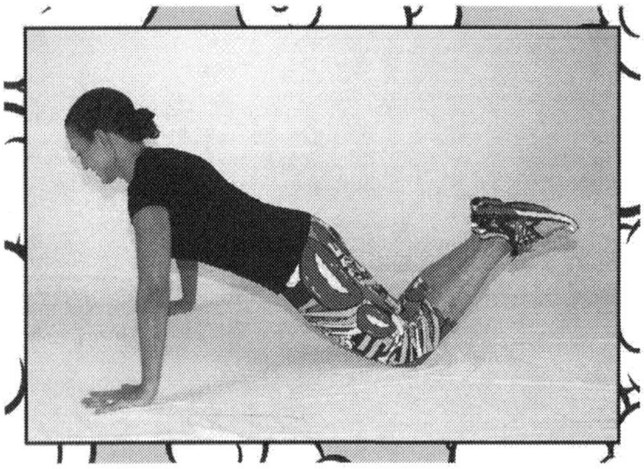

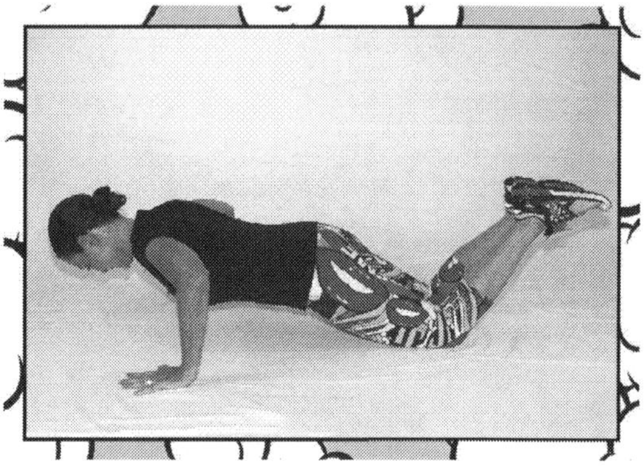

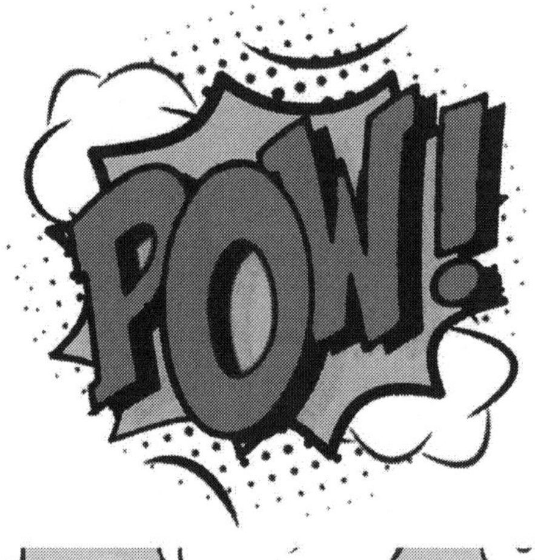

Advanced

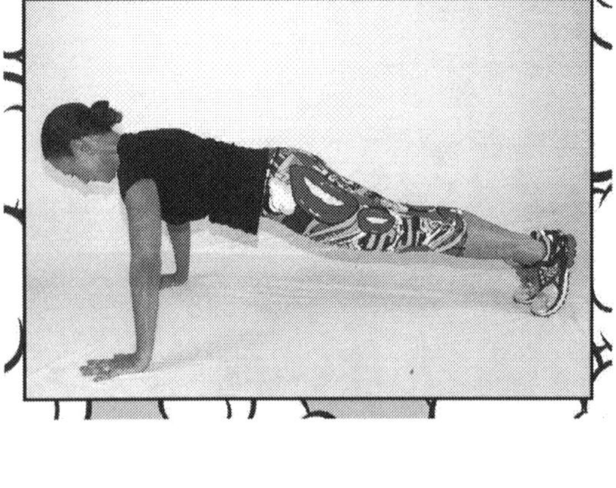

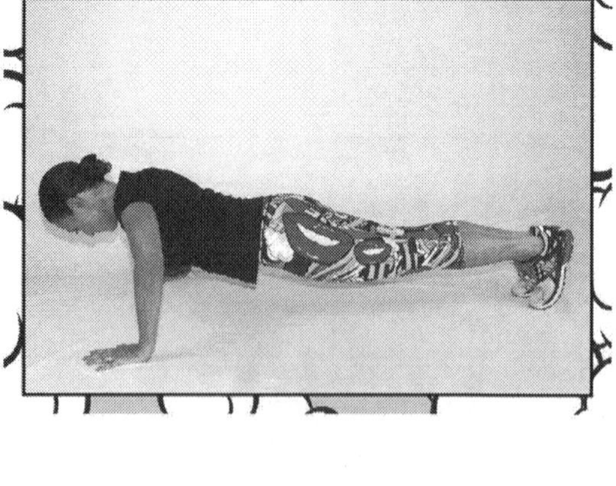

Side Plank Lie on your side and lift your body up onto your elbow. Extend your legs out placing the body weight on the outer edge of your feet. Hold the abdominals in tight and focus on your breathing.

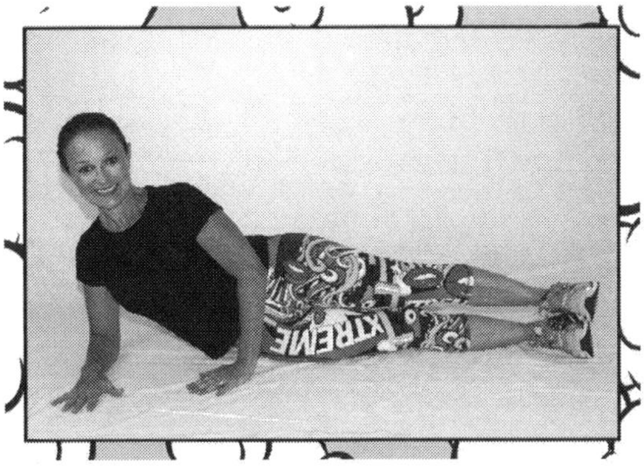

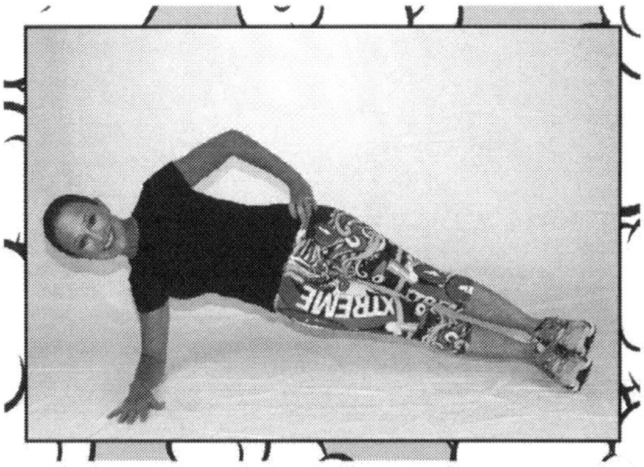

Bridge Lying on the floor, bend your knees and set your feet down hip width apart. Next, slowly begin to peel your spine up off the floor starting from your tail bone. Once you get up to your neck, slowly start to set your spine back down on the mat and repeat.

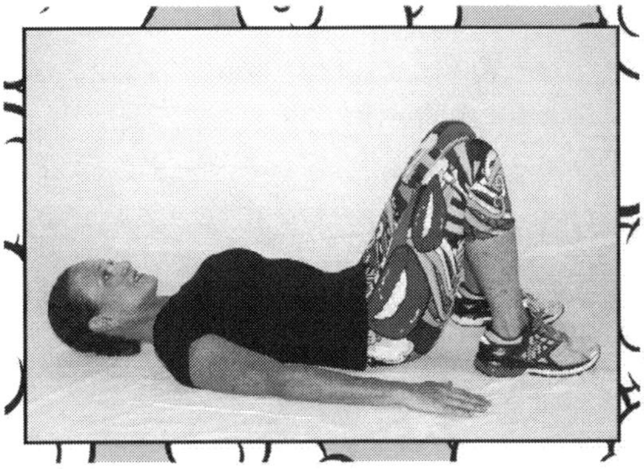

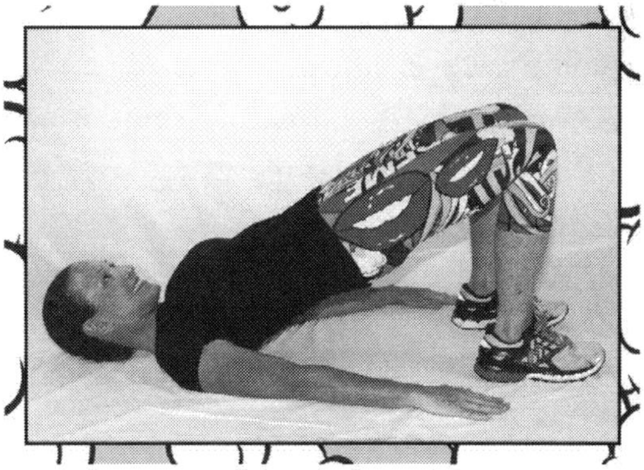

Crunches Abs are designed to stretch for pregnancy but stay flat for life. Crunches are best performed on your back with your knees bent and feet flat on the floor. Hands support the weight of the head and the rib cage contracts inward to force the head and upper body to come up and then down.

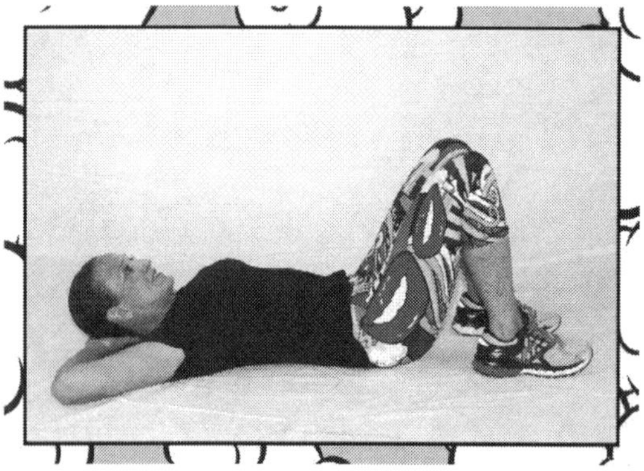

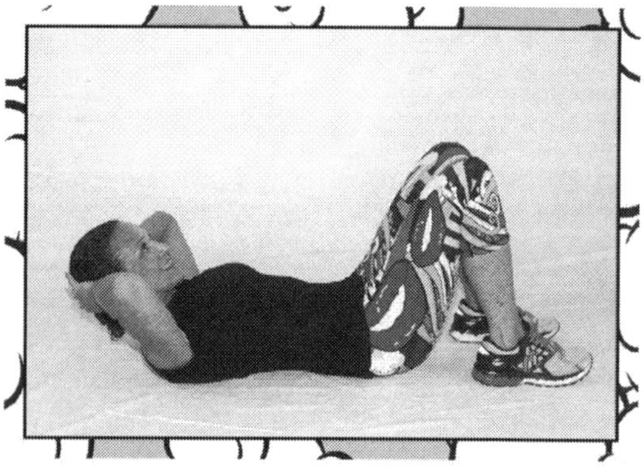

Leg Lowers From a lying down position, place your hands behind your head and hold yourself up in a high crunch. Next, extend both legs straight up above the hips and feel your spine pressed firmly into the floor. Keep the upper body in place and slowly lower your legs until you feel like your spine is about to arch (don't let it), then bring your legs back up and repeat. You can also do these with bent knees as a modification.

Advanced

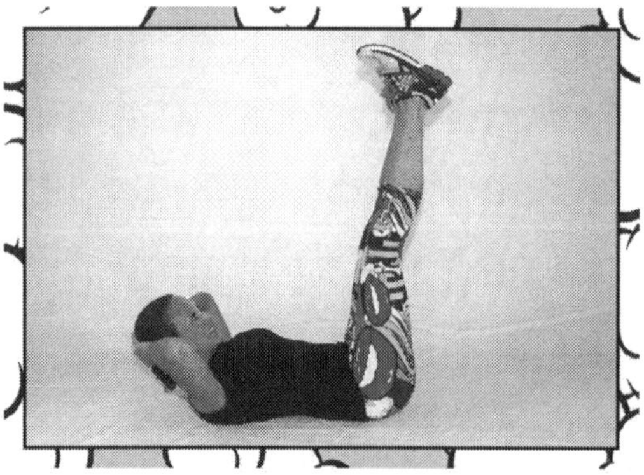

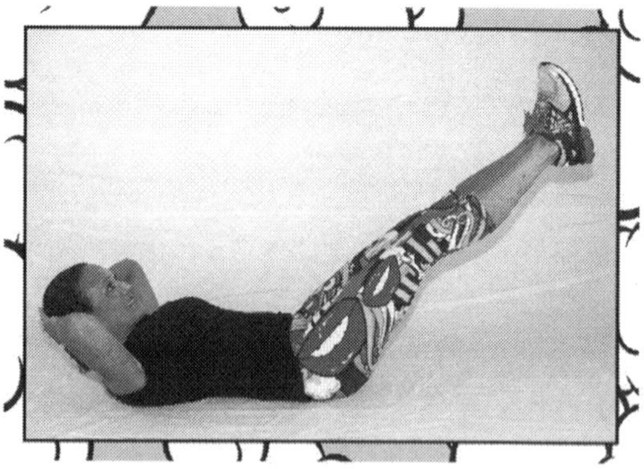

SUPER POWERS

RPE SCALE

PERCIEVED EXURTION

BURNING FAT WITH OXYGEN

KEEPING YOUR HEART RATE WITHIN YOUR IDEAL RANGE FOR CARDIOVASCULAR CONDITIONING

RPE 10
MAX EFFORT ACTIVITY
Feels like you have overdone it, you are toast! Completely out of breath, unable to talk, and sucking wind. You can not hold this pace for very long.

RPE 9
VERY HARD ACTIVITY
You are starting to gasp, you can barley speak and it is pretty hard to maintain this intensity.

RPE 7-8
VIGOROUS ACTIVITY
YOU ARE BURNING FAT!! It's a little uncomfortable, you can speak a clear sentence with just a little huff and puff in there.

RPE 4-6
MODERATE ACTIVITY
You feel like your working out. You are a bit uncomfortable, but it is doable. You can carry a conversation but in short bouts.

RPE 2-3
LIGHT ACTIVITY
You can speak clearly, gossip about whatever you want, and you feel like you could keep this pace for hours.

RPE 1
VERY LIGHT ACTIVITY
Your working harder than you would watching a soap opera on TV, or even sleeping. Not much happening here, you could easily do this for hours!

In order to BURN FAT you need oxygen!

You need to speak clearly, without Huffing and Puffing

But you need to work hard enough to almost get you to take that Huff!

SuperPower Cardio

How much is too much or not enough? That, my friend, is the question. So how do you figure it all out?

RPE (rate of perceived exertion) is used to gauge your intensity in your workouts. To burn the most fat, you want to be at a 7–8 every workout.

SUPERPOWER TIP: For those who don't want to step into a gym, not to worry, streaming videos are here. There are now these great online subscription services to keep you on track when you're not sure what you're doing or you're snowed in, this is the way to go. Check out the resource page at the back of the book for my "top picks".

SUPER POWERS Cardio

Here are my top 6 SUPERPOWER fat blasting moves.

Jacks Jumping Jacks pump the blood quick and strong. Both legs go out with a soft bend in the knees, arms up, and as the legs come back together, the arms go down.

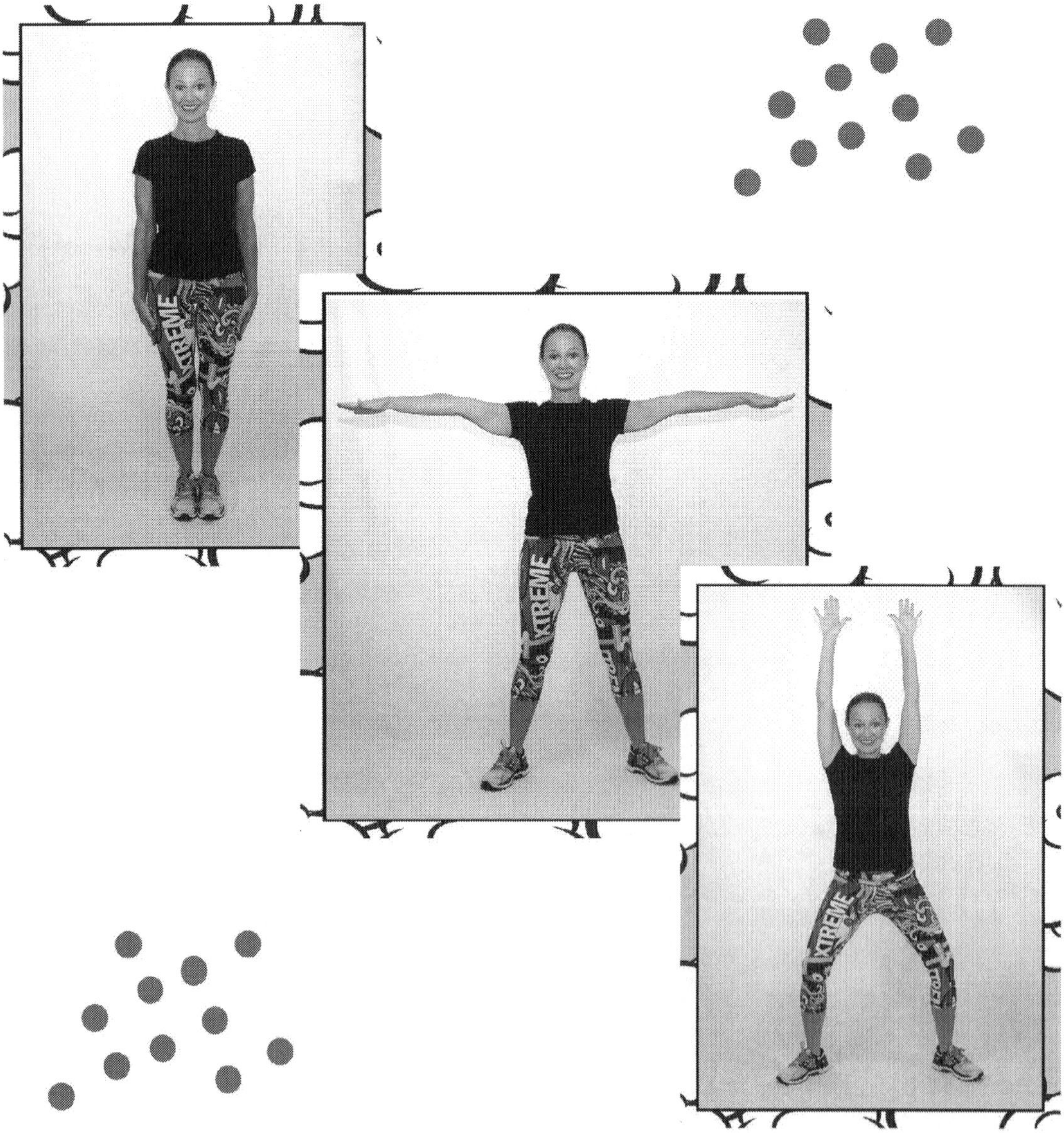

Just Dance Cardio is simple. The key is to increase your heart rate and break out into a sweat. So if you don't want to follow a choreographed routine, don't. Turn up the music and *shake your groove* anyway YOU want.

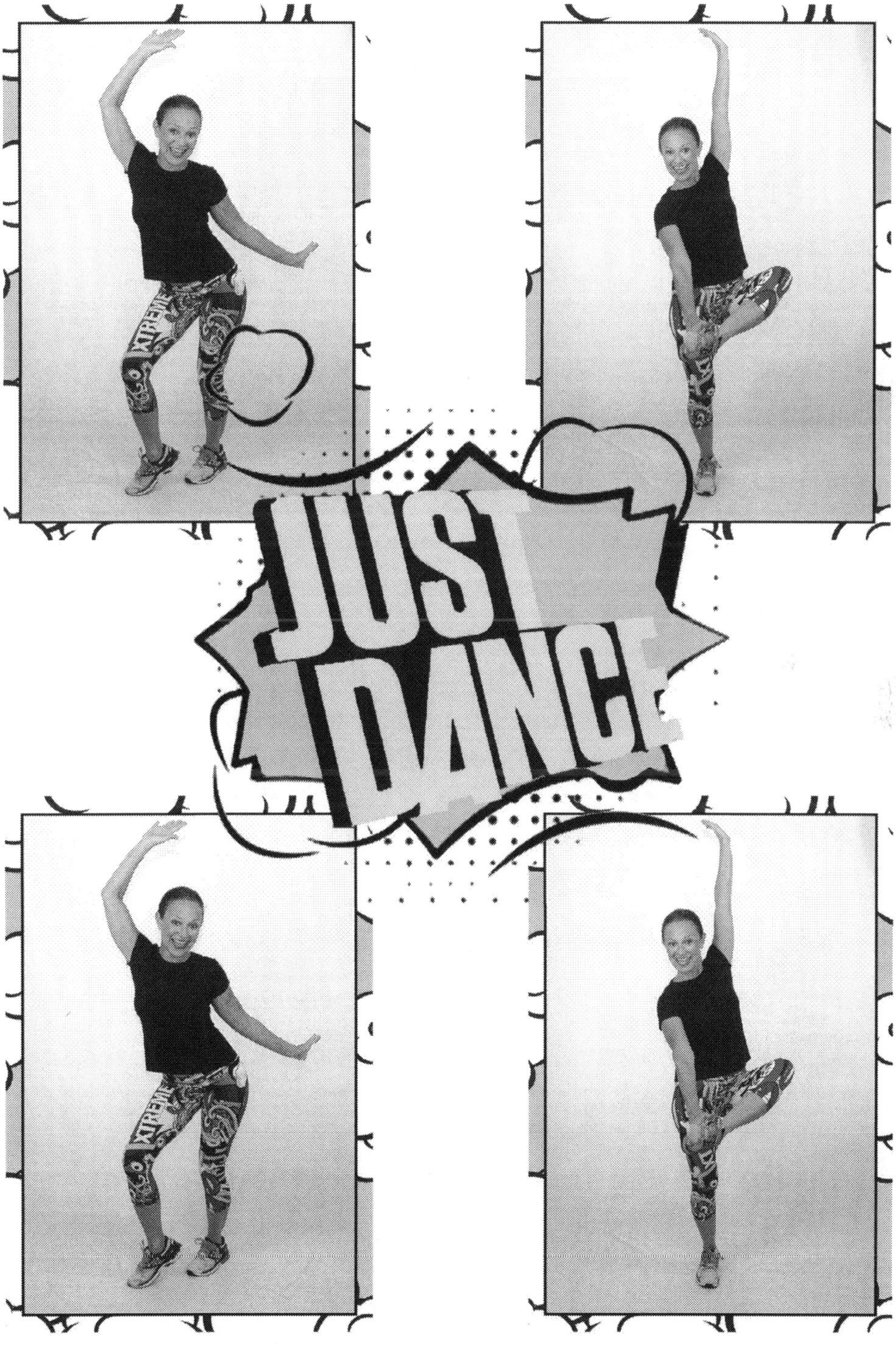

Scissor Jacks Get that bootie to kick in. Alternate your legs forward and back as if you are skiing, then add in your arms to give that heart rate an additional boost.

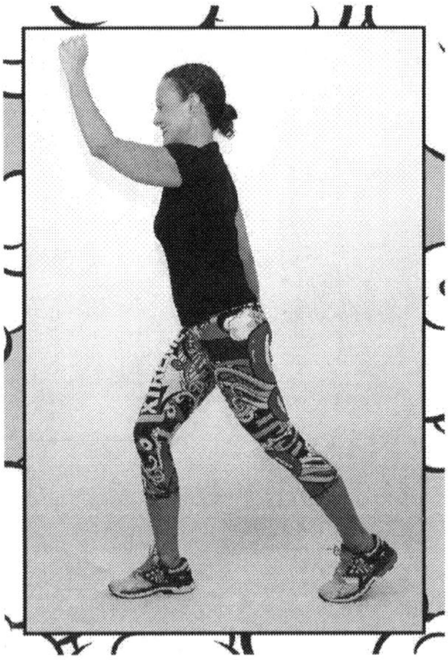

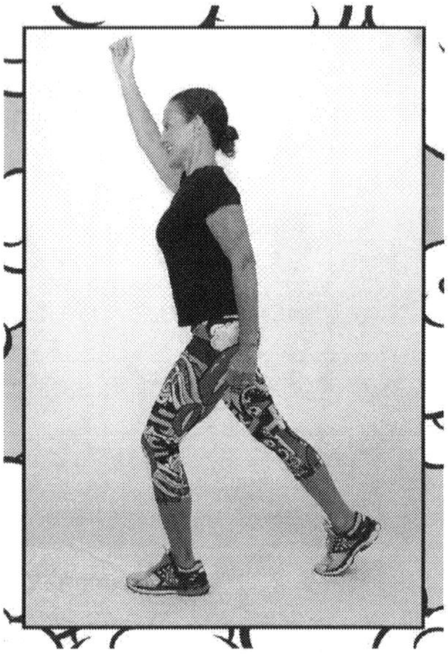

High Knees You are running in place. Picking up the knees increases the heart rate and definitely makes you *sweat*. The key is to land softly through the foot – toe, ball, heal.

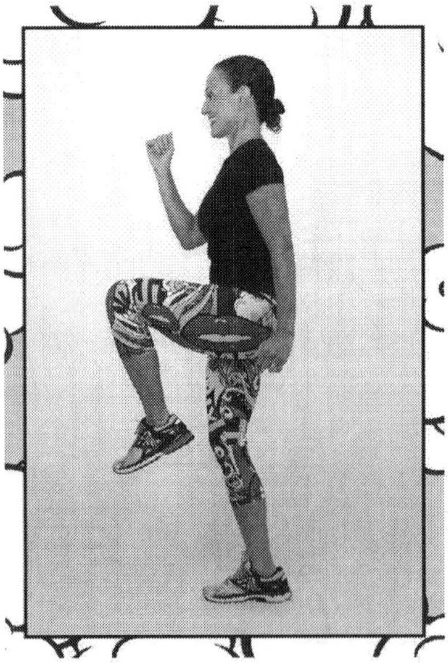

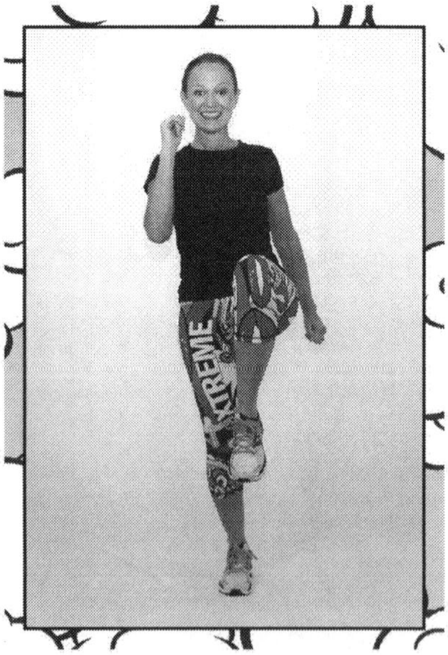

Jump Rope With a Jump Rope in hand, start to move the rope around. If you are a novice to jump rope, no worries, simply start my turning the rope on one side of the body. Once you have the rhythm of the rope then you can work on your jumps. It's all about practice.

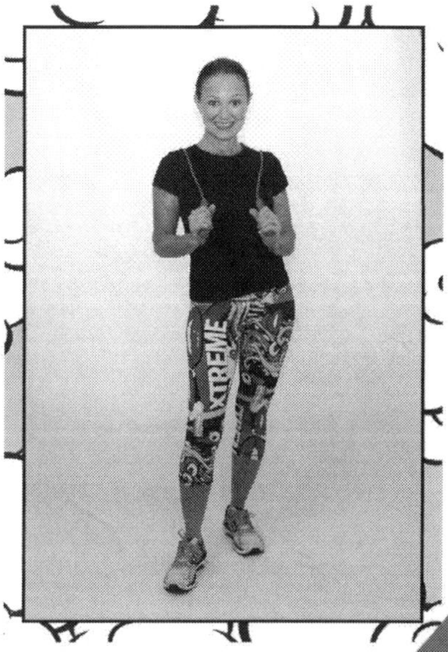

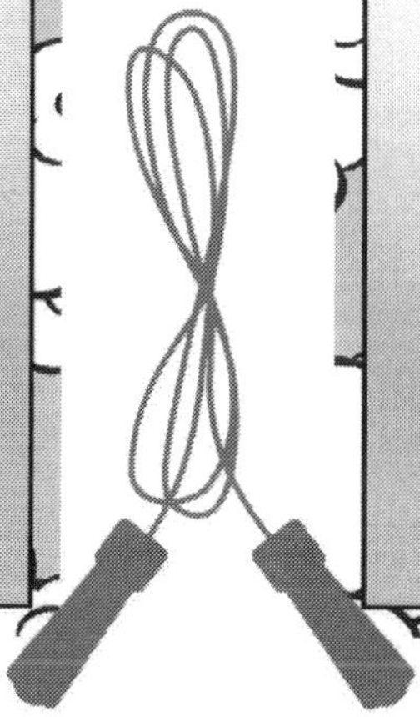

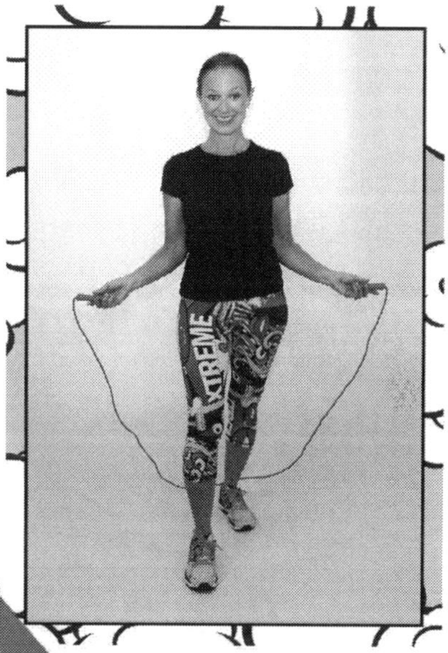

Running You can take this to the streets or keep it inside, just be sure your SuperPowers don't take you flying high! Land softly through your feet and keep your posture upright and abdominals held in tight.

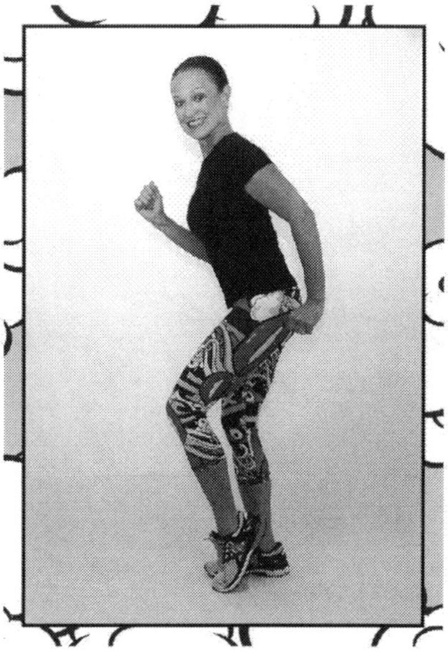

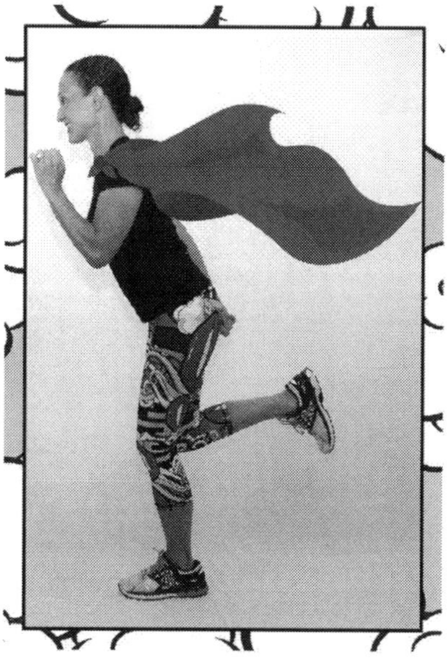

SUPER POWERS Stretches

Here are my 3 favorite SUPERPOWER stretches.

Butterfly Take a seat and bring the soles of your feet together. Allow your knees to lower to the floor or mat. Not to worry if your knees are up or down, just allow the stretch from your hips. Work on sitting up as straight as you can, with the chest high, and the shoulders back and down. Then give yourself a slight lean forward and feel your inner thigh beg for forgiveness.

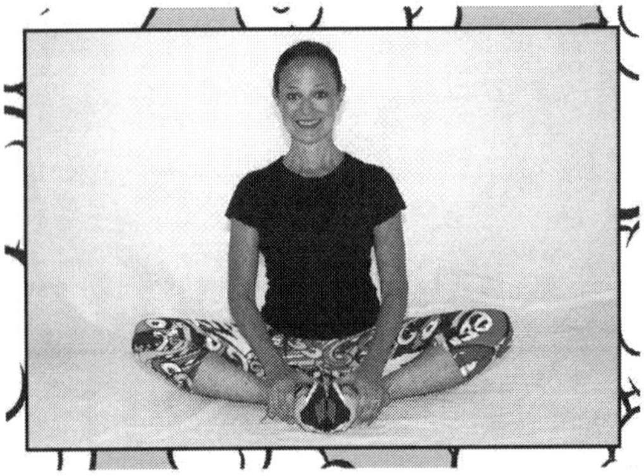

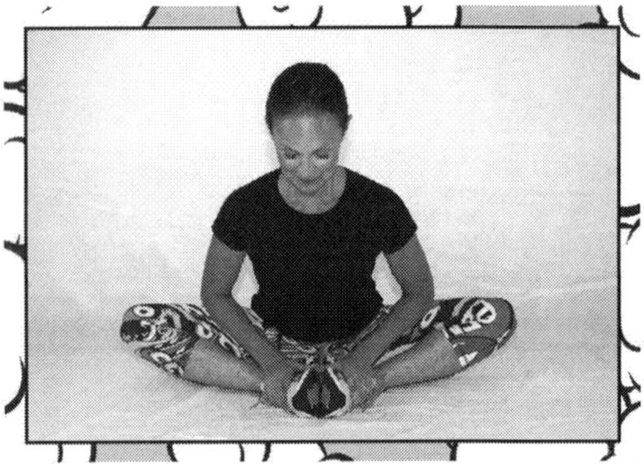

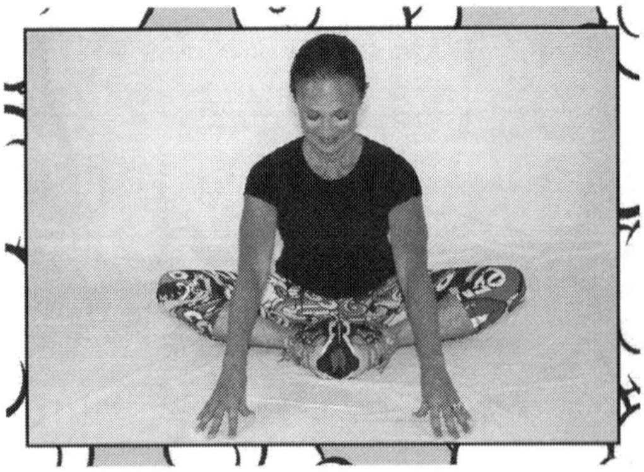

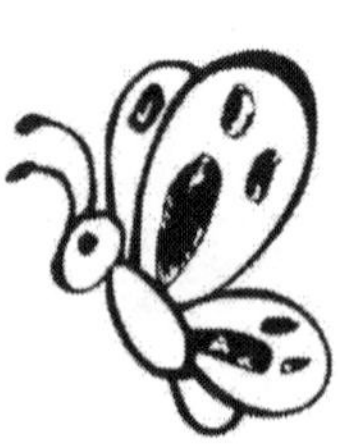

Side Stretch Remaining in a seated position, place one leg out to the side and bend the other foot into the center. Moving towards the straight leg, bend your body sideways, still maintaining the chest up and the shoulder back and experience the stretch right along the side of the body.

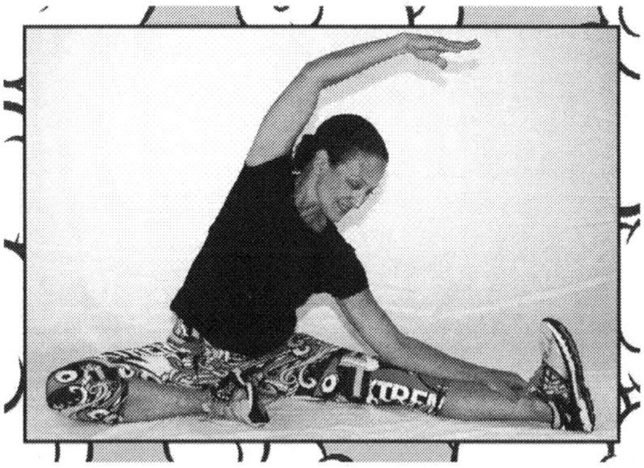

Forward Bend Now, place both legs out in front of you. Set your spine upright with the shoulders back and lean forward from the center of the chest. You can do this with your arms straight out. As you lean forward from the hip joint, you will feel the stretch along the back side of your legs.

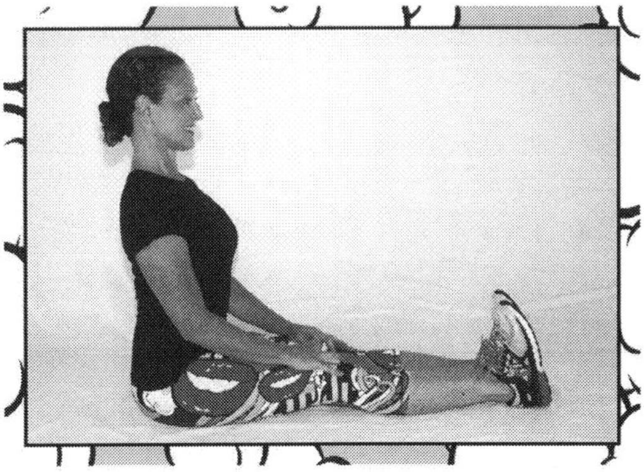

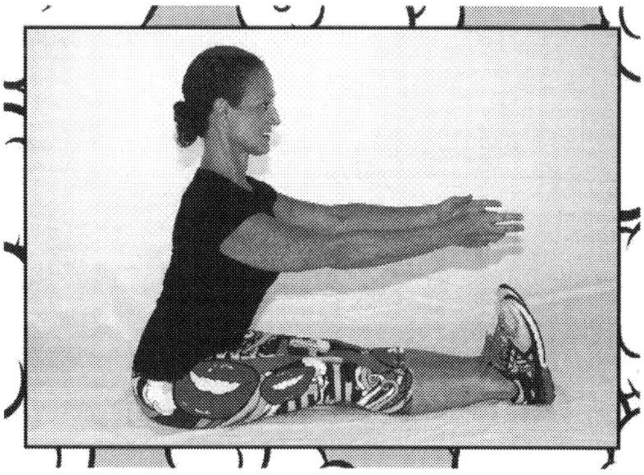

10-15 min Workout Routines

Exercise may not always be easy, but once you get your system down it will become part of your daily routine. To get you started, here are a few of my favorites. You can squeeze parts of them in for an easy 10–15 minute workout; don't let time be your barrier!

For the unmotivated, let's give this a try: I want you to set aside 10–15 minutes (and actually 5 would do just as well), that's right, not too long, not too short. So for that time here's your task, first let's start with music, something fun that you enjoy for dancing, singing or grooving to. Next, there is no real equipment needed except for a towel, mat or rug. Here's your workout, feel free to try it all or break it into tiny pieces so they can fit neatly into your day. And if it still feels too overwhelming, go to the end of this book in the ***Fitting It All In*** section and follow the 8-week plan.

- 5 minutes of freestyle dancing, set the timer on your phone or clock
- Stretch – Sit with the legs out in front, back straight and bend forward from the hip. Hold for 25 sec. then do the same thing with the soles of the feet together as in a butterfly stretch
- 10 pushups
- 10 squats
- 5 minutes of freestyle dancing
- 10 lunges
- 10 crunches
- 5 minutes of freestyle dancing
- 5 pushups
- 5 squats
- 5 lunges
- 5 crunches
- Stretch your way to the finish line! Same stretches as above, also add some side bending stretches and arm stretches

Now, once you have mastered that one, or if you're a bit more regimented, here's a good one that also requires no equipment and can easily be done in your house, park or neighbor's yard.

It's a calorie burning Interval Training. This workout incorporates 30 seconds of activity with 30 seconds of rest, although for most of you this rest really isn't rest, it just sounds good. You will have 6 intervals, each interval you will do 1–4 times. Now, granted if you need a true rest you can add in a one-minute break in between intervals (for this minute you can drink water, walk in circles or just suck wind so you're ready for the next one).

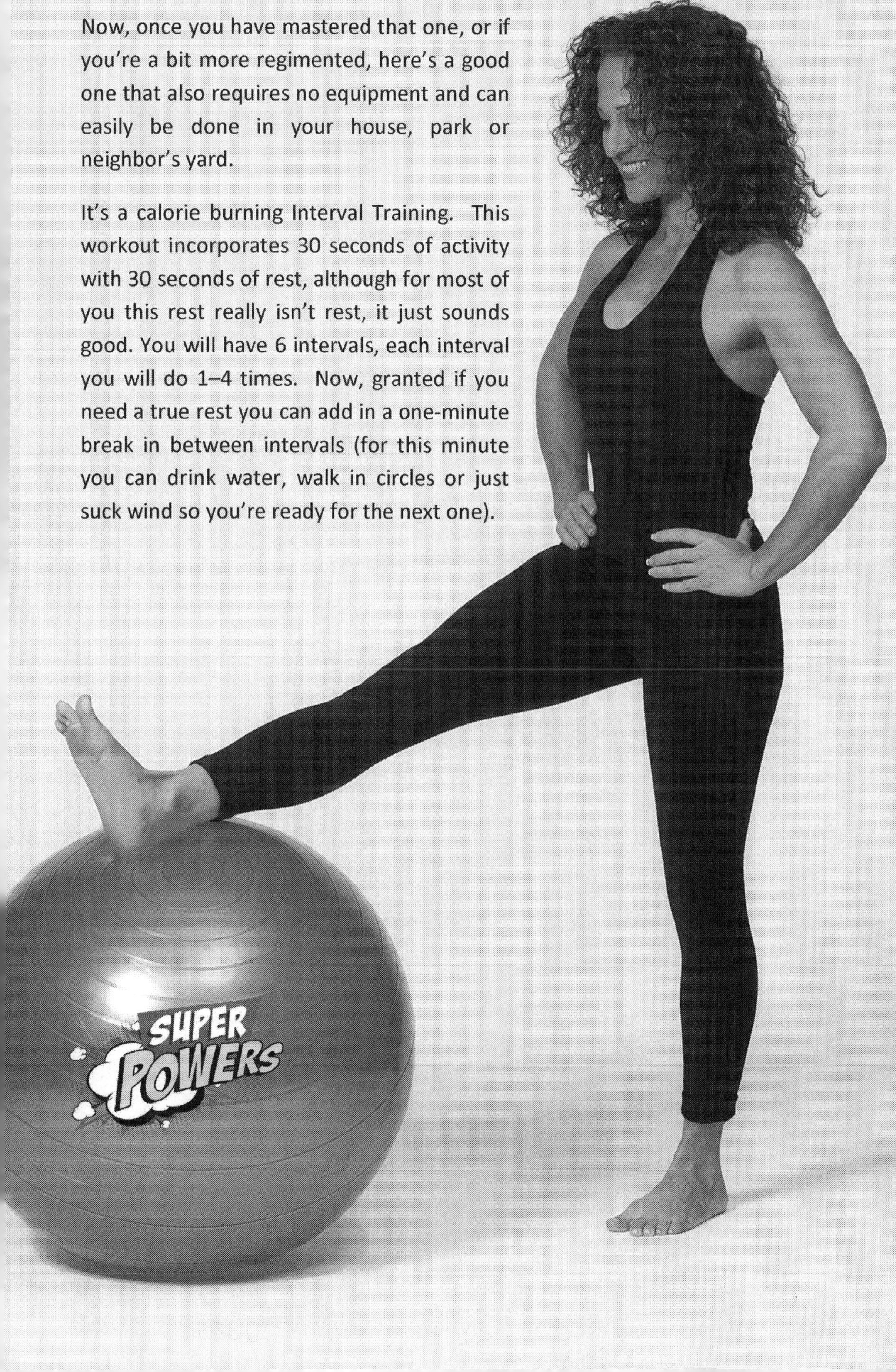

SUPER POWERS Calorie Burning Interval Training

A= Active and R=Rest, well not really rest, it's more like active rest!

Interval 1	Interval 2	Interval 3
A Jump Rope (either with a real rope or a pretend one, whichever works) R Push Ups	A Jumping Jacks R Squats	A Running in Place R Abdominal Crunches

Interval 4	Interval 5	Interval 6
A Jump Rope R Lunges	A Running with Knees High R Leg Lowers	A Scissor Jacks R Abdominals

A & R should be done for 30 seconds each

Time Cruncher
Do 1 repetition of each interval if limited on time.

Hard Core
Take each interval and repeat 2 - 4 times before moving on to the next one.

At the End
Stretch for 2 minutes

Listen, I realize some of you love this stuff and others would prefer a root canal, but one thing is for sure; our bodies were designed to move and deserve the benefits of strength and endurance from those movements. You have two choices, ramp up your day-to-day chores and hobbies to rev up your heart rate and sweat or find an exercise schedule that works for you. You may have to do a bit of homework and figure out the right class, program, trainer or hobby that gets your heart rate going and your body moving each and every day, but trust me, it is doable!

Track your progress like a pro!

Whether it is a watch, a smartphone or whichever gadget you enjoy using, make it work for you. Think of it as your personal body monitor. Here are some wonderful things Dr. Daniel Virgil, professor at The David Geffen School of Medicine at UCLA, found to help you understand your ups and downs a bit better:

During your day to day: Your heart rate is a wonderful assistant that teaches you how you're doing. What do I mean by that? Your heart rate will change if you are stressed, dehydrated, you're starting to get sick, or maybe you have lied to the boss, either way you will see a change in your day-to-day heart rate, so keep a look out!

On a week-to-week basis – If you have increased your activity and been following the plan, your daily heart rate might be lower; yup, lower than usual because you are getting fitter and your heart is more efficient. Relish and enjoy this!

During sleep, as you will come to learn, your body both mentally and physically recovers. If you check your pulse from the night before and notice that your heart rate rose 15 or more bpm several times throughout the night ... hmmm. You are not sleeping well and receiving the benefits that you totally deserve. This will zap your SuperPowers and leave you frazzled.

SUPERPOWER TIP: SuperPowers flourish with the right care and maintenance. Move the body right, and yes it will get tight, but it will also give you extra hours in your day, and ramp up your endorphins for that "feel good" type feeling.

"Recovery brings us to center, balances our energy, and inspires us for all of the greatness ahead"

-Adita Lang♡

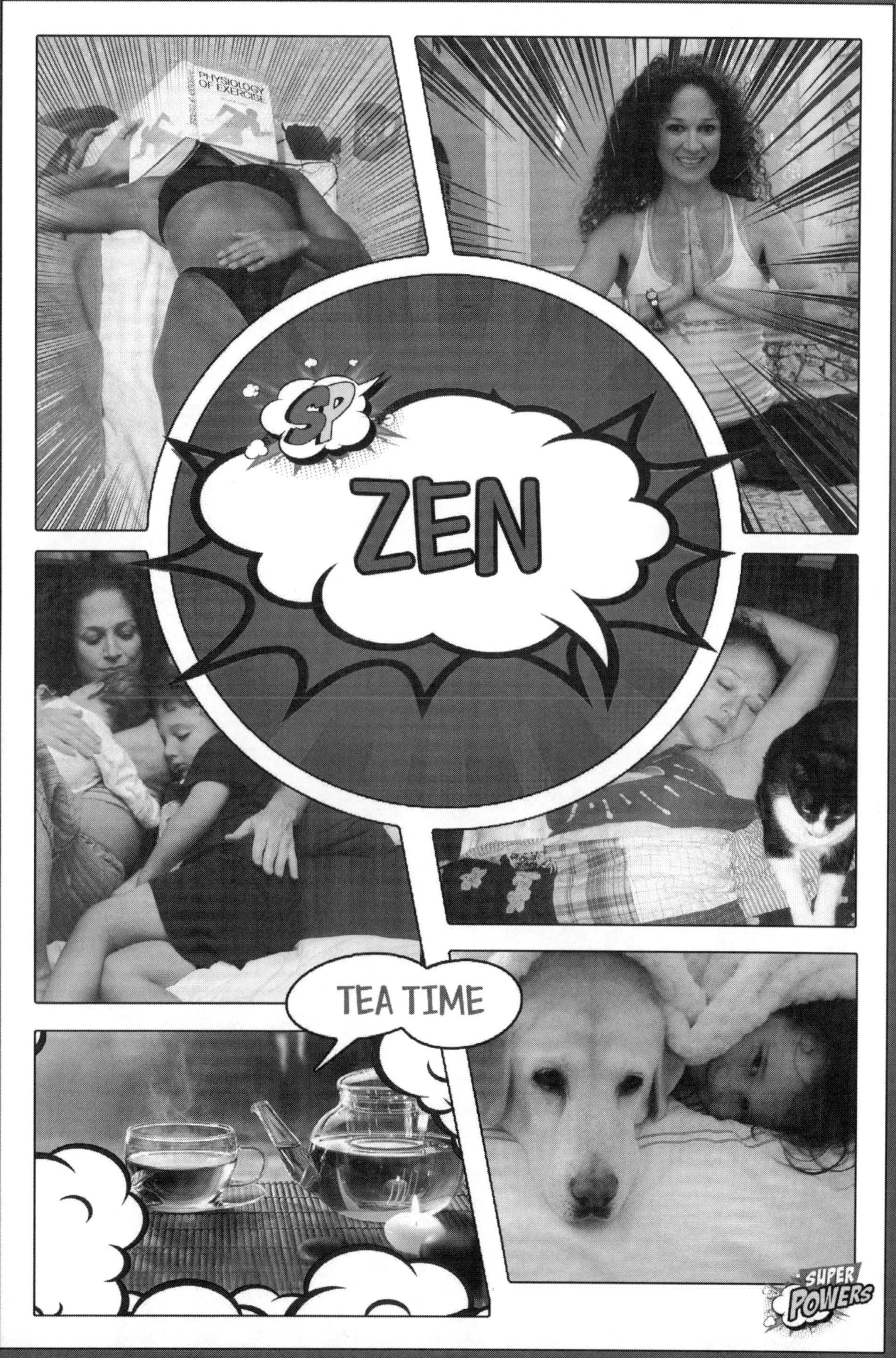
PHYSIOLOGY OF EXERCISE
SP
ZEN
TEA TIME
SUPER POWERS

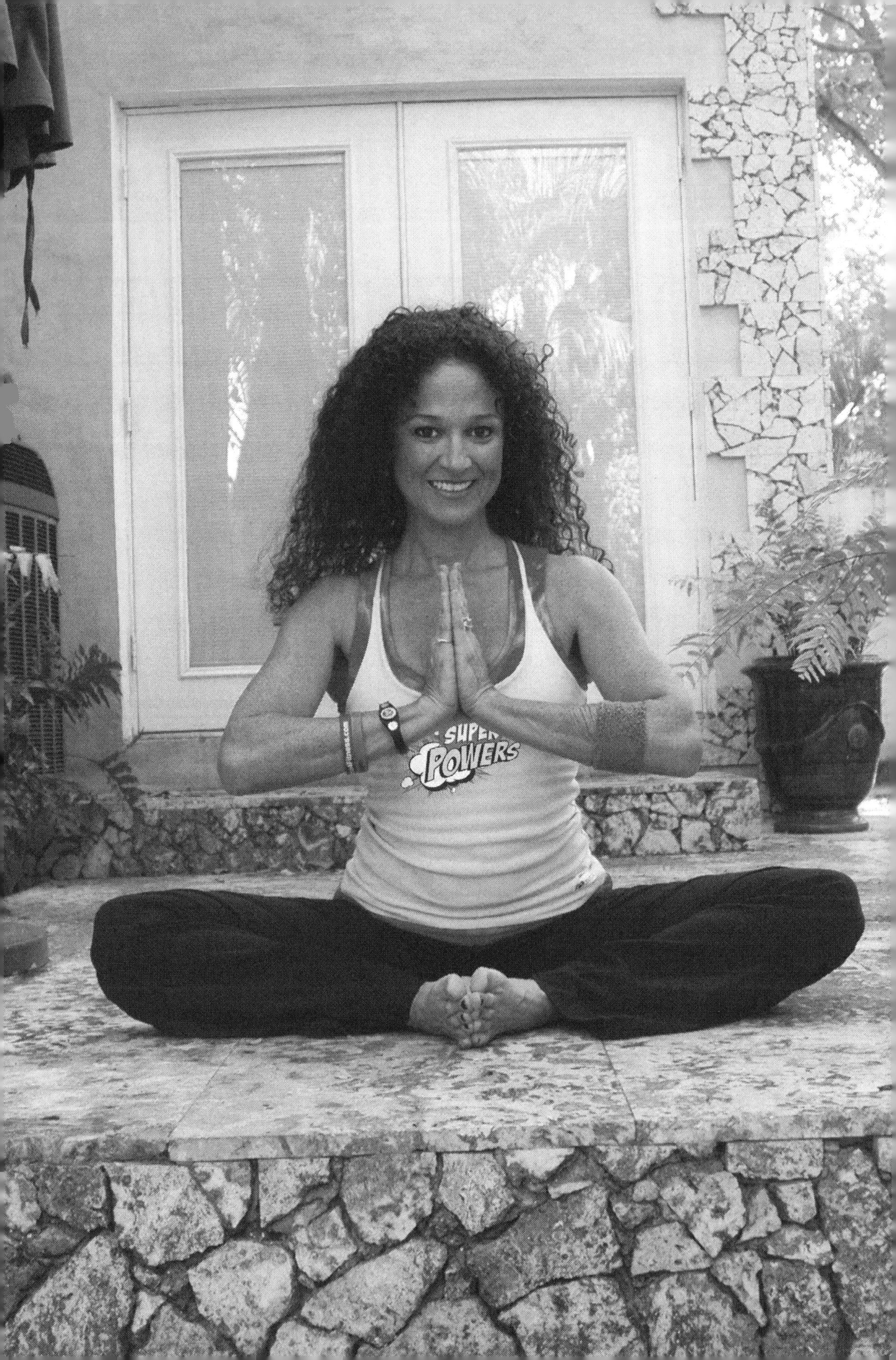
SUPER
POWERS

The Zen of SuperPowers

Sleep and Relaxation

A woman with SuperPowers is the ultimate of full-time jobs, and many SuperWomen even layer several jobs on top of that one. Some people out there say that "sleep is not that big of a deal" and "when we die we will get all the sleep we need anyways," well, they must not be SuperWomen, we need sleep and that is all there is to it. Sleep helps us combat stress, lose weight, and recharges our system for the next day of adventures and chaos. The old me lived for the party and still made it to teach my 7 a.m. class. A nap was a bonus but never a prerequisite. The new me tried living on survival mode, but that was short-lived. My SuperPowers became SuperGrumpy and my multitasking, type-A personality training became fuzzier than ever. Have you ever started something and halfway through you forgot what it was that you were doing? Oh ya, brain fog at its best! We need RECOVERY people, and the only way to do that is through Sleep and Relaxation.

Amazingly enough, sleep plays a major role in how quickly our bodies adjust and change. Ideally our sleep patterns would mimic those of the sun and moon, realistically that will never happen with a schedule like ours! So our next best thing is to understand how our bodies function with rest and incorporate it as much as possible in order to reap the benefits.

Cortisol *(red line)*: Think of this as our "daytime booster", a hormone manufactured in the adrenal glands. With normal sleep, cortisol is recharged during sleep and will naturally decline throughout the day and lead us back into amazing sleep. This hormone is directly involved in the metabolism of carbohydrates and influences our levels of glucose available for activity and energy; in other words, when it is not working right, it can make us FAT and LAZY! It puts up an anti-stress shield but can be easily depleted with too much stress, leaving us too pooped to pop.

Serotonin *(blue line)*: Here's our "sleepy guy", a neurotransmitter that multitasks at its best but has a big involvement in your mood, appetite, and sleep. With normal sleep patterns, serotonin kicks in at night, during sleep, and helps to repair and rejuvenate the muscles and the mind (which, of course, I can always use). Serotonin levels are affected by specific foods, nutrients and exercise—the more muscle one has the more serotonin is produced and the better we sleep and recuperate. Don't forget to lift heavy things, my friends!

These are the two main components that help to provide us with sufficient rest, recuperation, and energy for our next big marathon of the day. Cortisol and serotonin cannot work at the same time. Cortisol is active during the day—light wakes it up and helps to energize us; on the other hand, serotonin kicks in with darkness and brings us into a deep slumber. The key to optimal rest is to recognize that during the stage of serotonin any light that comes to us will wake up cortisol and disrupt our sleep. Once disrupted, or if disrupted throughout the night, this will then affect our physical and mental recuperation. With this said, it's important to sleep in a pitch-dark room, you may need to block out small LED lights or change the brightness on your clock, but true darkness is the winner here.

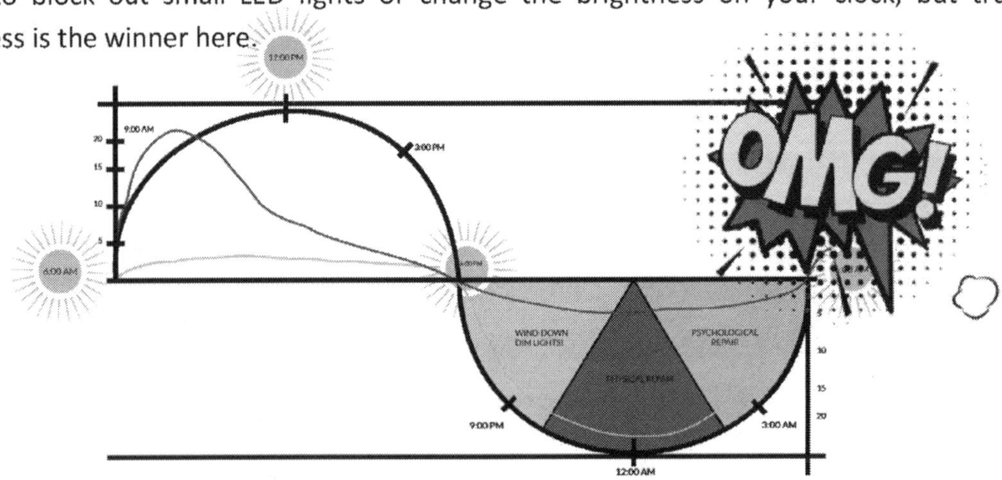

When our bodies sleep, we recover from all of it, every bit of stress, exhaustion, and chaos we have put ourselves through. This is the time for our bodies to recharge in order for us to ... do it all over again. So here it is in a nutshell:

10:00 p.m. – 2:00 a.m. – Physical Repair: This is when our bodies recuperate from all of the physical activity, running around and stress we put on our bodies throughout the day. This is when our muscles develop, grow stronger, and repair from any damage.

2:00 a.m. – 6:00 a.m. – Psychological Repair: This is when all of our thoughts, stresses, and emotions receive a "time out" to disappear, forgive or just chill, and our mind gets a chance to rejuvenate from all of it.

If you constantly go to bed late, your body will not repair appropriately and your physical gains will take forever. On the flip side, if you are constantly getting up way too early, your mind doesn't have a chance to truly relax. This leaves you stressed with the ability to bite off the head of anyone who gets in your way and leaves you with little energy to do the things that you really want to do.

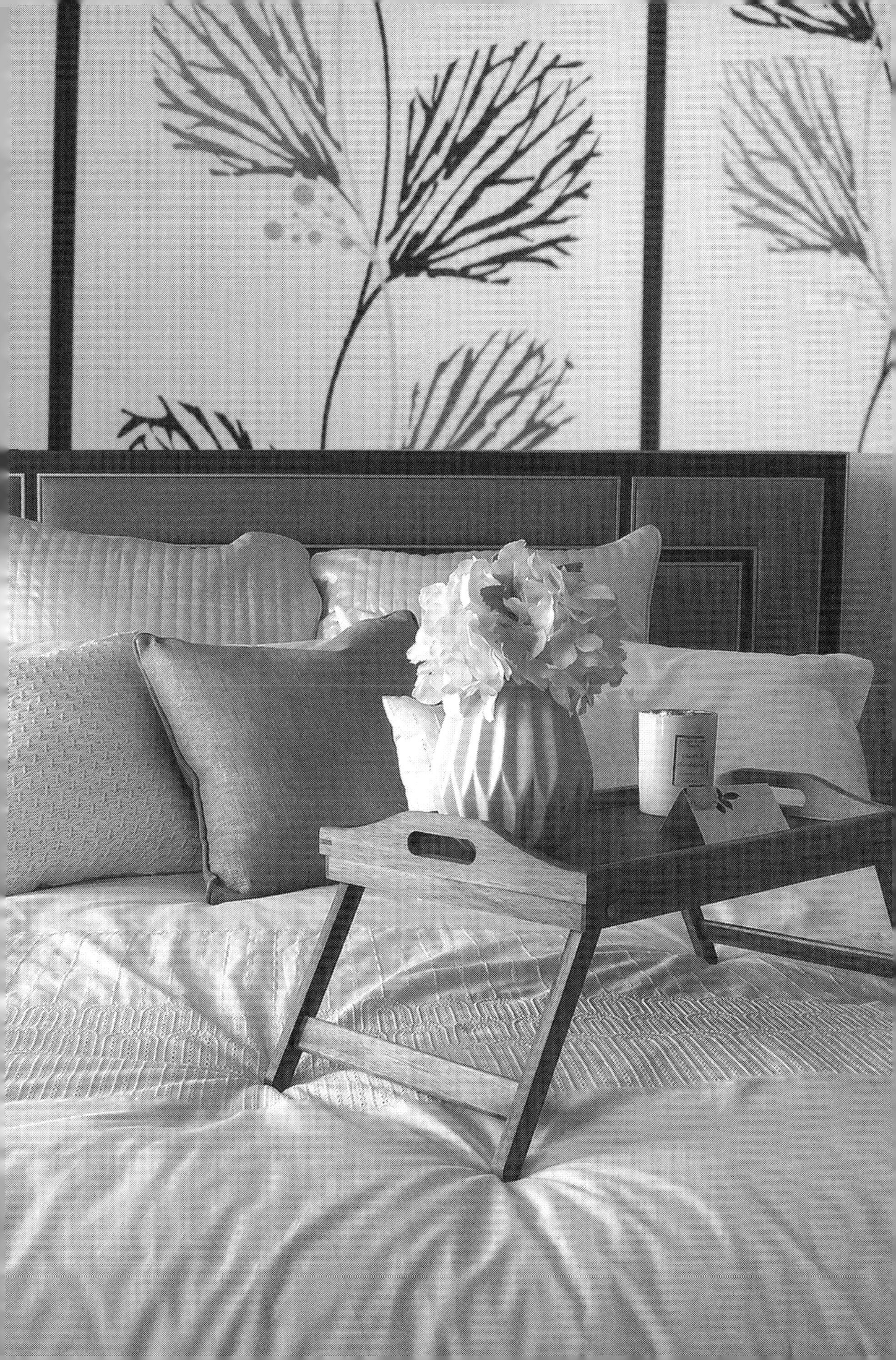

As crazy as this may seem, this is very closely interrelated to one's success. We all have our own baggage at home, and life gets crazy, but you are the only one who can take care of YOU. These Four Pillars all work together and each is just as important as the next. By you taking the steps to maximize your health, your SuperWoman abilities will gain more strength and power than ever before. We can't just "survive" on a few hours of sleep; this does no one any good, not those around you and not you. So if you have challenges with sleep I want you to take a real good look at your nighttime rituals. You can't move from maximum overload right into sleep, it's like a great wine, you need to slowly work your way to it to reap all of the benefits it brings. Here are a few things to enhance your "Z" making slumber that can make it much more peaceful:

1. Take a survey of your room at night – Is it totally dark? Can you cover up any light that comes in? Is the temperature cool enough?

2. What is your nighttime ritual? Are you watching action-packed adventures before drifting off or are you relaxing with a cup of tea and a book?

3. There are a ton of tea options to help you unwind and doze off, try them out and find one you really enjoy. (*chamomile, lavender, and kava*)

4. Your room should be your retreat sanctuary, get rid of the boxes, papers, and any additional work stuff that only reminds you of the things that have to get done. You want to enter your room as the one place where there is nothing more that needs to get done, no laundry, no tasks, simply sleep and... (well, you know what I mean).

5. There are also several apps that will dim the screen of your phone or tablet by removing or dimming the blue light. This is the light on your favorite gadget that causes sleep disturbances and keeps you awake.

6. No caffeine or exercise within 3 hours of shuteye time; there is no need to ramp up your energy at this time!

7. And if there are other sleep disturbances you have not addressed, get it done, sleep is way too important to miss out on.

A good nighttime ritual in a soothing space can give you hours of extra energy and laughter in your day—it's totally worth it! Now, just as important as your nighttime rituals, are your daytime "relaxers". Only YOU can create a schedule and environment that propels your SuperPowers to a whole new level. Part of that is choosing the right relaxation tools to use during your typical day and even to do some "double time" when the hamster wheel you are on just won't STOP! For some people religion takes them away from the chaos and recharges the soul, others need something a bit different. Either way your soul needs a constant flow of TLC to keep us at peace and at ease. Find what works best for you, let your inner guide enjoy quality time with you and watch how all of the chaos of your day just seems a bit less chaotic than you thought!

Relaxation Rituals...

Take a notebook and on each page write something that is relaxing and enjoyable to you. Then on those days when the "overwhelm" takes over, open your notebook randomly to a page, and do whatever is on that page for as long a period of time as you have available to you.

Meditation

This one took me a long, long time to accept, but I am so glad I have added it into my repertoire. Meditation is so much more than sitting in a knotted position looking for enlightenment, it's about shutting off the world for just a few moments so that your thoughts can unravel and your mind can take a break. There are more ways to meditate than you can imagine. We all have days filled with so many "To-Do's", but they will still be there even if you take a 10-minute time out. Filling up our day is easy, stopping for just a brief moment seems to be the challenge of the day, but guess what ... it's OK to stop, the world will go on and you will still finish your infamous "to-do" list. This is about "self-care" and taking that brief moment to just "pay attention". You can do this waiting at a doctor's office, sitting in traffic or just stopping for a scheduled 10 minutes, whatever works, but once you start you will find this becomes a very important part of your day. Even if you think I'm nuts, it won't hurt to try this, so see what happens...

Here are a few of my favorites, choose one and try it out for at least four days. Think of it this way, the first day you try it, it's new, it's different, so you're not that good at it. The next time you try, you're more familiar, it's a bit easier. Then, by the fourth time, you can really have a feel of what it's all about. By this time you can decide if you have chosen the right thing for you, if not choose another one until one just clicks.

1. Guided Meditation – Having a voice from an audio or video guides you into deep relaxation. I'm pretty picky, it's got to be a good voice with a good message, but feel free to experiment. There are apps, YouTube videos, and tons of resources available to try from.
2. Julia Cameron, Morning Pages – This is such an amazing practice. Basically, take 3 pages in a notebook and simply write. Write anything that comes to mind, complete sentences or not, there are no rules, it's a huge "mind dump", letting it all out. It's a great way to create new ideas, elaborate on old ones or mumble your way through. Oh wait, there is one more rule, they have to be handwritten and you MUST complete all three pages.
3. Coloring in a Coloring Book – Yes, you heard it right, this is a great way to shut the world out and use your creativity or non-creativity to bring you back to center. And guess what. Feel free to color in the lines or out, no one will grade you and no one will judge!
4. Deepak Chopra's Free 21-Day Meditations – Deepak and Oprah have come together to offer some amazing guided meditations. These are offered a few times a year and are a great way to either start your new practice or enhance your existing one.

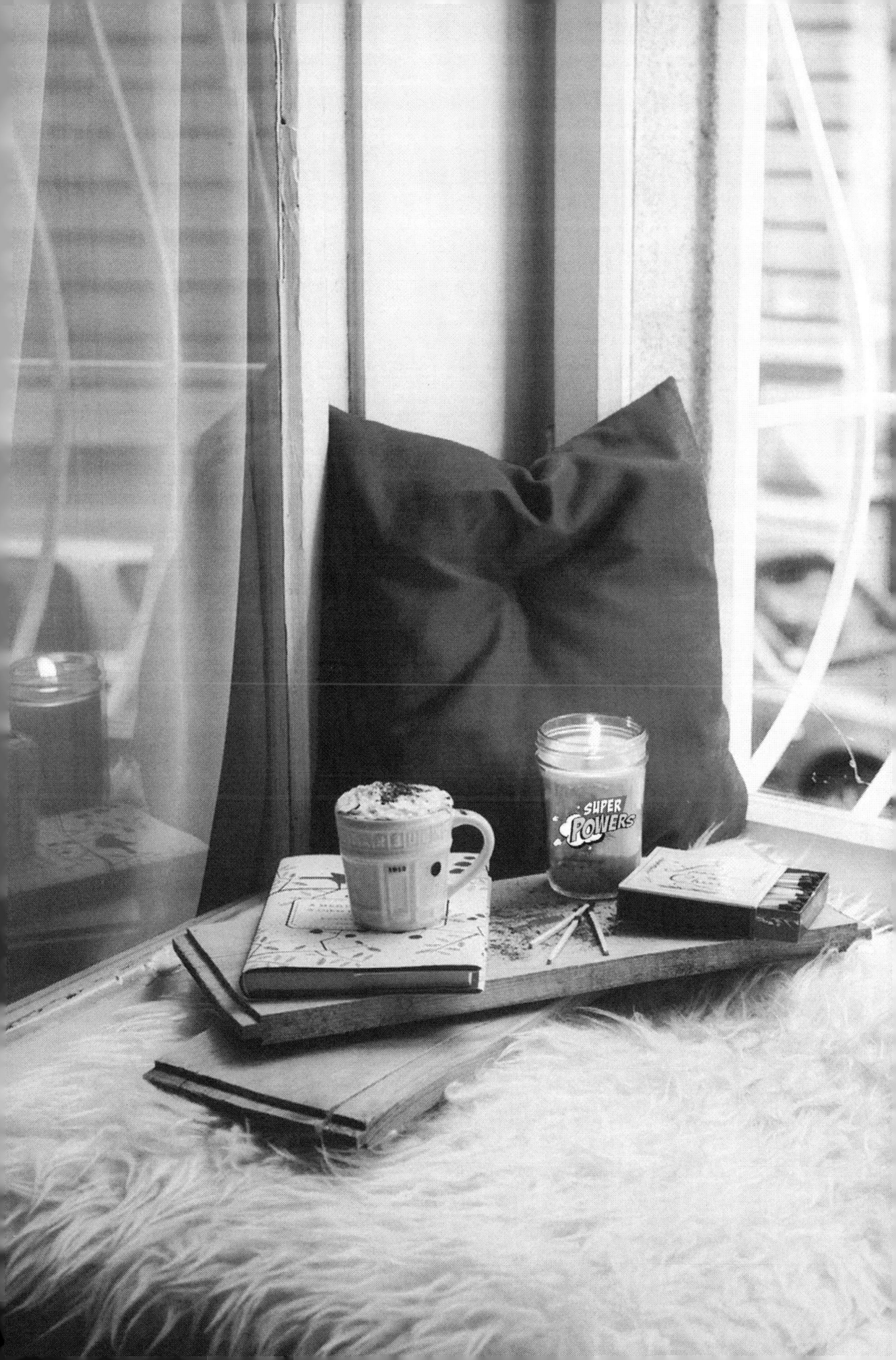
SUPER
POWERS

5. Anything that requires very little brain power and that you can truly focus on can become your meditation. Who knew that gardening, ironing or simply beading a necklace could give you your Zen? Focus on your breath with each and every movement and allow little space to think of anything else. Enjoy it!

6. Focused Meditation – This is where you simply focus on something. It could be the flame of a candle, the sound of your breath or the sound of a soothing vibration or bell. My favorite focused meditation is concentrating on the length of my breath, so try these...

Meditations from 1–10 minutes (you control the time)

- Sitting or lying down, close your eyes and simply count as you inhale and count as you exhale. Your goal is to extend your inhale and your exhale as much as you can. You may start out by getting to the number 7 and then you progressively get to 10 or more. Set an alarm if you want to try to do it for 5–10 minutes or you can even try doing it for 8 or more breathing cycles, whatever works.

- Sitting or lying down, close your eyes and inhale to a count of four and then hold the breath in to a count of 4. Next exhale to a count of four and hold for an additional count of four and repeat the entire thing again. You can either decide how many of these you will do or set a time, whichever works best.

- Lying down, start by taking in two deep breaths; for the next inhale point your toes as hard as you can and, as you exhale, let it go. Inhale and now tighten up your thighs (quadriceps), and as you exhale, let it go. Inhale and tighten up your glutes (tush, boodie, you know, your back end) and exhale, and let it go. Inhale and tighten up your abdominals, and as you exhale, let it go. Inhale and pull back and tighten your shoulder blades together and exhale, and let it go. Inhale and push your arms down, and exhale and let it go. Inhale and pull your shoulders to your ears and exhale, and let it go. Now simply breathe and feel the entire body relaxed. If there is an area that stays tight, breathe into it and let it go. Take a few more deep breaths and give yourself a positive affirmation before getting up!

Wake Up Rituals **Breakfast** Mid-Day

The Best Saturday EVER!!

Design your most amazing day ever,
write it out with tons of detail and make it happen.

Fun Stuff Relaxation Rituals ***Activity*** **Dinner**

The Best Night Ever ____________________

It's All About ME!

Official Membership Form for

____

What are your 10 most common ME time favorites?

1.
2.
3.
4.
5.
6.
7.
8.
9.
10.

These should be things that you could do any day of the week!

How many minutes per day can I count on ME for at least one of these?

SuperPowers with a Smile Roadmap: 20 ways to spend an hour

1. ______________________________
2. ______________________________
3. ______________________________
4. ______________________________
5. ______________________________
6. ______________________________
7. ______________________________
8. ______________________________
9. ______________________________
10. ______________________________
11. ______________________________
12. ______________________________
13. ______________________________
14. ______________________________
15. ______________________________
16. ______________________________
17. ______________________________
18. ______________________________
19. ______________________________
20. ______________________________

SuperCharge your day!

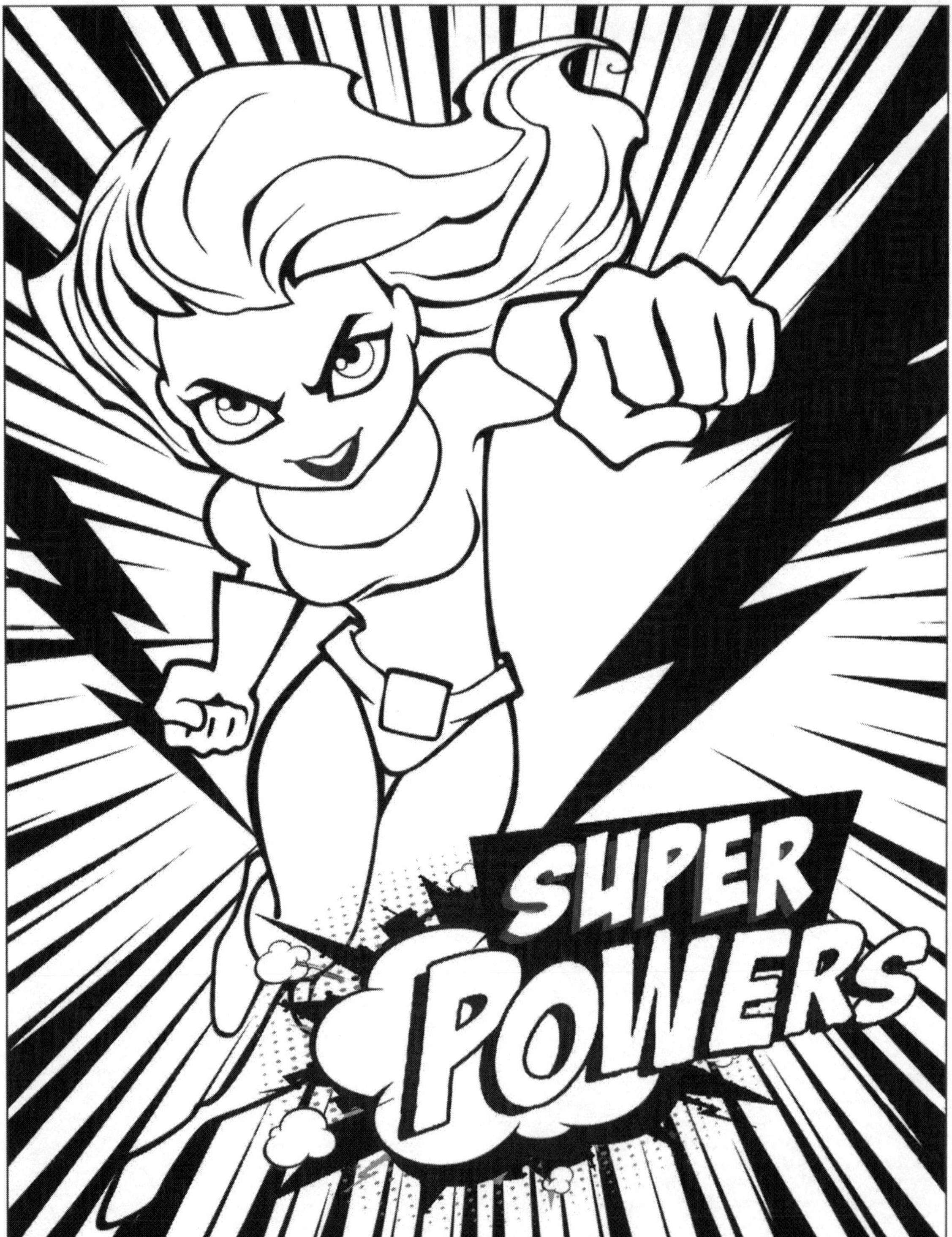

Color me in.

Color me in and relax.

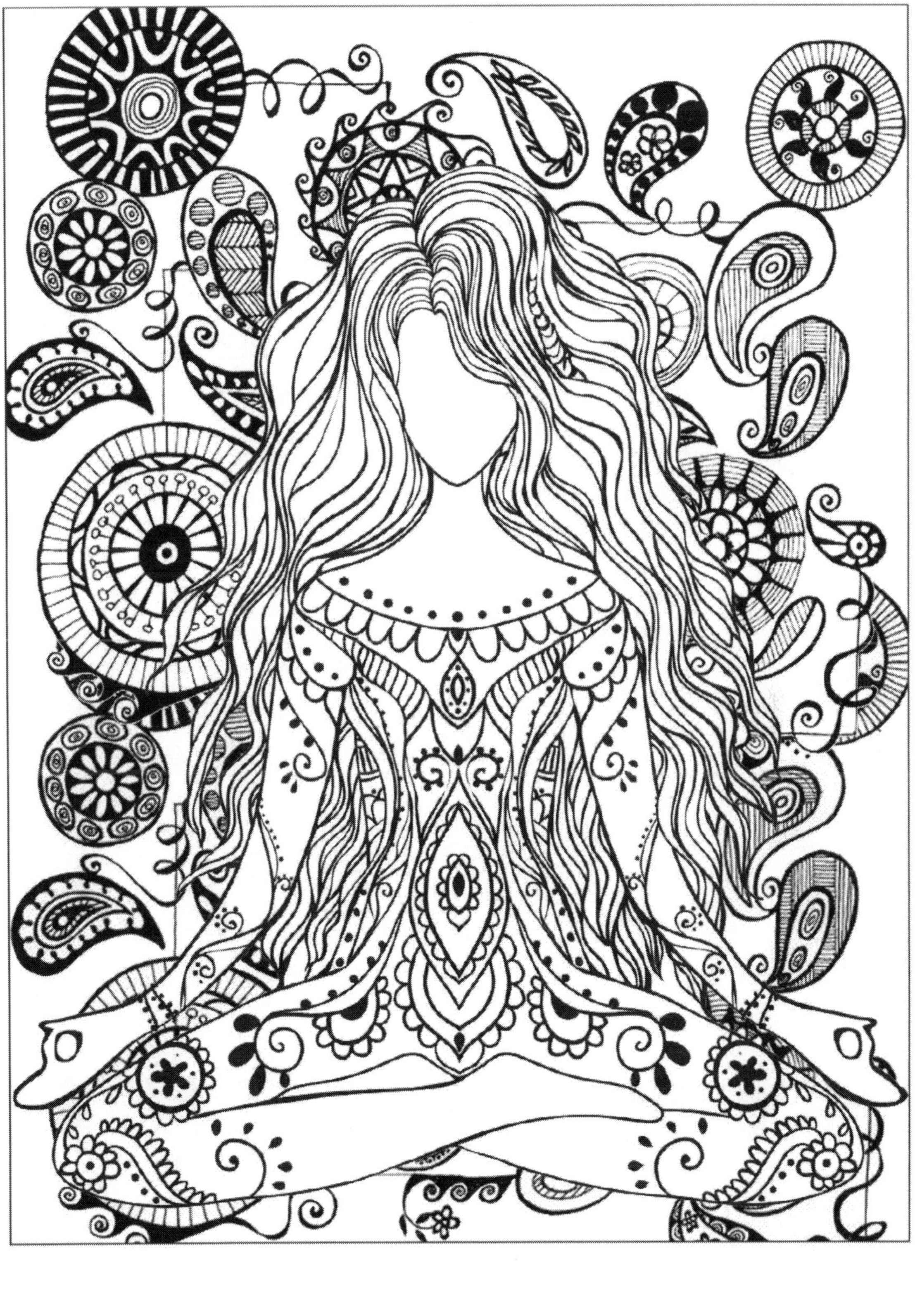

"Anyone can laugh, but
when you laugh so deeply
that the tears pour out, the
body ignites with radiating joy
that it becomes contagious"

-Adita Lang ♡

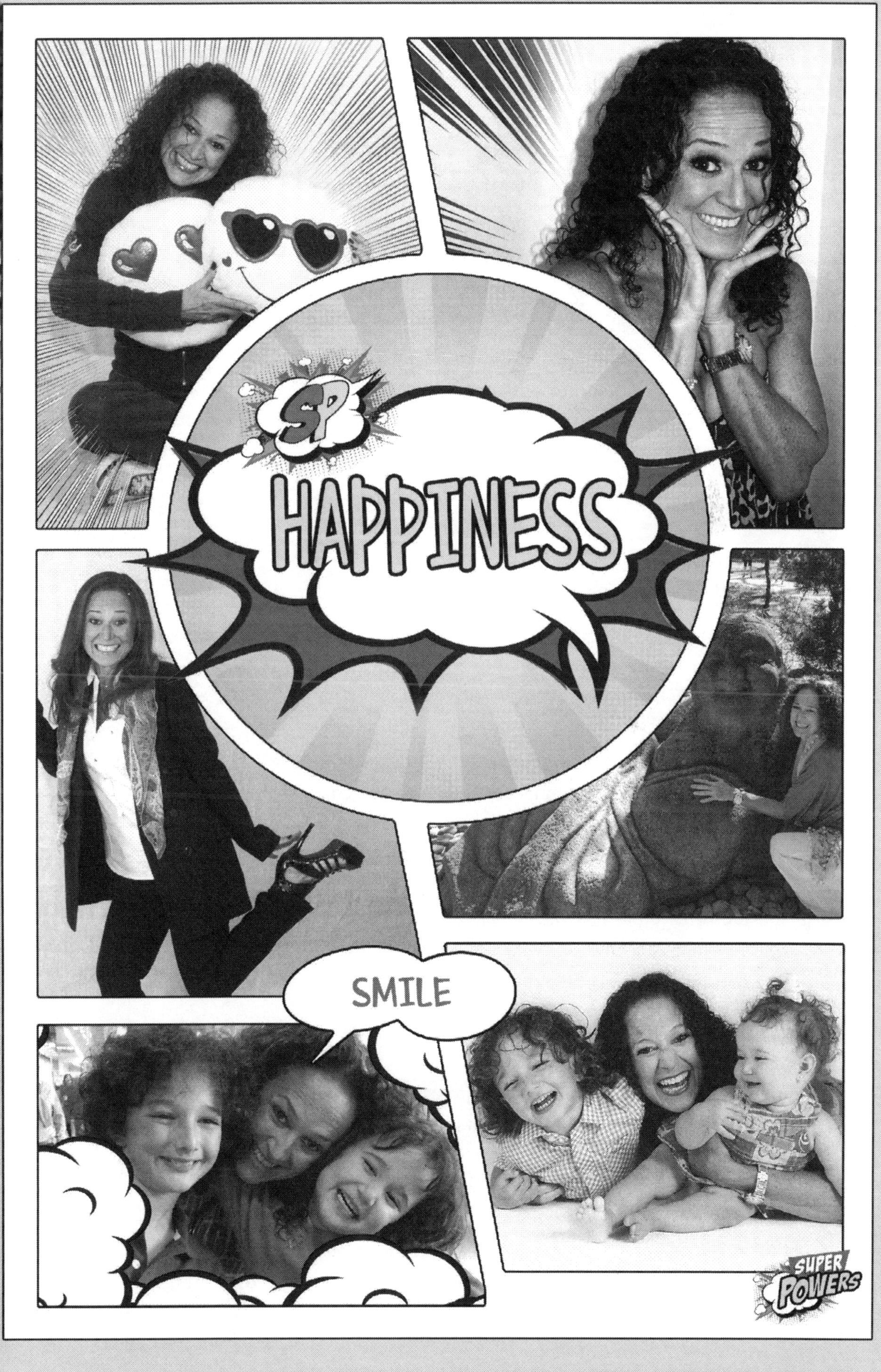
SP
HAPPINESS
SMILE
SUPER POWERS

SuperPowers with a Smile

Happiness

Yes, life's enjoyment also plays a pivotal role in your health... Who knew? Making it a priority to enjoy as much as you can in your day to day has a huge impact when combined with the other four pillars. Without happiness we cannot motivate and encourage others to be their very best, we lose drive and enthusiasm, resulting in sluggishness, lethargy and women with SuperPowers who have lost their ability to fly. Life is meant to be enjoyed and personal satisfaction and gain come from our purpose for living and the aspirations that drive us to be our very best. It's time to release the perfectionism and just "let go" and enjoy, make happiness one of your top priorities. You control your schedule and you control everything that you are putting on your plate (even if someone else puts it on your plate!), so make a plan to include at least one thing that gives you a huge smile on your face each and every day, make a date with the girls or just make a call to catch up—you know what does it, so put it into action!

I was SPOILED, when fitness was my full-time gig, I was surrounded by fun and immature colleagues; we took responsibility seriously but in a light and carefree type of a way with laughter as our drug of choice. Once I entered the MOTHERHOOD arena, there were way too many responsibilities, sleepless nights, and fellow moms that were living on survival mode as well. Laughter became about a few day-to-day events but caffeine became more important. The endorphins from both exercise and laughter clear out the mind and give us an outlook of complete enjoyment. As your fourth pillar, this is as important as the other three, if not sometimes more. Happiness is something that comes from within, it makes you feel alive and well, we can't allow those around us to "rain on our parade".

Think of it this way, when you are truly happy from the inside, you shine a bright light that lights the way for so many others!

We Only Live Once! *At least in this lifetime!*

Here are a few things to consider that life coach Barry Gotlied shared one day:

- Avoid the news, say "*No,*" to television, radio, and negative publications
- Don't condemn, criticize or complain ... become a solution finder instead
- Get rid of the "*Negatrons*" in your life – surround yourself with positive people
- Look for and share stories about positive people and events
- Share them with your family and friends
- Have an attitude of gratitude
- Read something inspirational, educational or spiritual each day
- Replace your limiting beliefs and fears with new, positive, empowering beliefs
- Take ownership of your life, seize the moment!

It's about focusing on the positive and minimizing the negatives. Remember, what we see or what is placed in front of us creates happiness and challenges or we are totally indifferent to it. This is because of how we interpret it, so if you're grumpy you will have a grumpy reaction to something that could be totally amazing. It's about making it a priority to laugh each and every day. Surround yourself with others who inspire and encourage you to be your very best. As the saying goes, "If you want to lose weight, eat lunch with your skinny friends." So if you want to increase your happiness, hang out with your "happy friends" and make yourself one of those "happy" people that others love to be with.

Everything in your life is your choice, you have the choice to listen, absorb or walk away. Responsibility for one's life is one of the hardest concepts to grasp, not because we don't understand it but because it's much easier to blame others for our challenges. Take a moment and consciously take note of the things you tend to blame others for. Now choose one of those things and think about another solution if you could not blame anyone for it. (For example, I gain weight because my husband wants to drink wine every night—you have the choice to drink wine or not, so the weight gain is not his fault, it is yours) This makes things a bit harder, some mental cleansing may need to happen, but in the long run it will make you a happier and healthier person for yourself and for those around you. You are a woman with SuperPowers, a force not to be reckoned with; there is no need to do things that you really don't want to in order to please a friend or two. Listen, if they are really your friends in the first place, they will be there no matter if you go to the fundraiser or not. I would much prefer to go laugh with a couple of girlfriends about silly stuff than be forced to make small talk with a bunch of yipidy yips. Do you remember the last time you laughed so hard that you cried? OMG these are my favorites. I start laughing so hard I can't stop, no matter what. I might make a few people crazy, but I sure feel great for the rest of the day from it. Or when was the last time you went to the movies and just started laughing out loud? Do it, girl, it's an endorphin overload that is worth every kooky look you might get.

Think back, when was the last time you laughed so hard you almost . . . peed in your pants? Write it here -

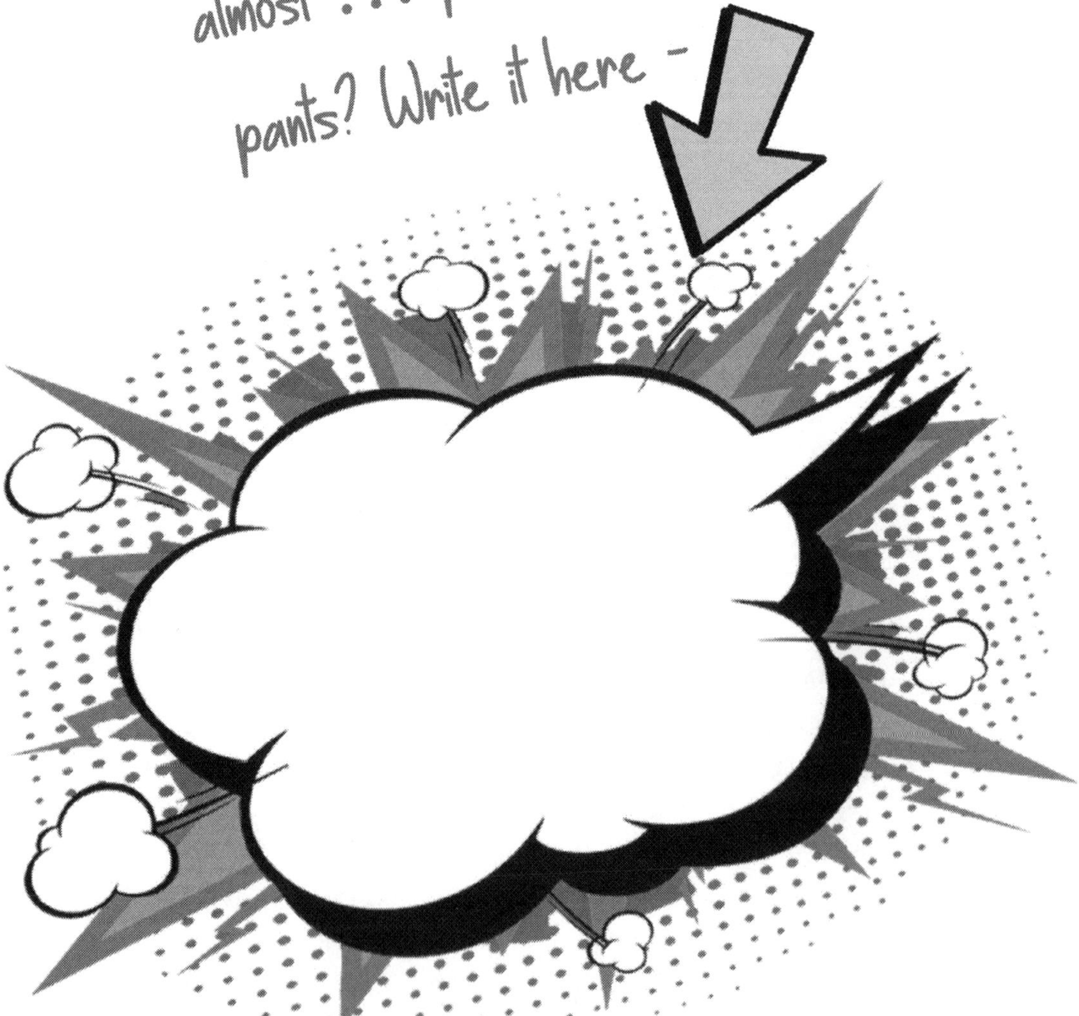

Best Friend Appreciation Page

To those amazing people in my life who do not judge me, criticize me, always look out for my best interests, and inspire me to be my very best... I salute YOU! You are a pillar in my world, we may or may not see each other on a day-to-day basis, but we always seem to reunite just at the right time. I THANK YOU for being a part of my life during the good times and during the bad ones as well.

BFF with Good Humor

BFF with Inspiration

BFF Mentor

BFF...Just Because

When you are truly at your Happiest...

How do you FEEL? Try using 5 different words to describe this:

____

____

____

____

How is your ENERGY? Try using 5 different words to describe this:

____

____

____

____

What other things do you experience? I know it's tricky, but try to find 5 more words, different from the ones above, to describe this:

____

____

____

____

How to Turn a BAD Situation Around!

As women with SuperPowers we can also easily become SuperFrustrated. We try hard to keep everyone at peace, on task, and everything in order, but sometimes it all unravels and we become more challenged than ever. For these moments of frustration, anger, and just plain old "pissed off" we need to have something to bring us back, clear our vision, and bring the "happy" back in. I have found that my shortness in temper and tolerance is that much more amplified when I'm hungry or tired, so for me a cup of tea and my 8 hours of sleep is a must to keep me on point. Now, granted, this is not always possible, but we each have to find that "thing" to bring us back to "happy". Here are a few things that have helped me minimize my frustrated moments and helped to amplify the happy ones:

1. No one can make us angry or frustrated, the reality is that we allow ourselves to get this way. We need to find a way to step back for even the slightest moment and look at the entire situation as a third party. Ya, at the time this probably sounds insane, but it can be done and the more you work at it the better you'll do. We all have to take responsibility for our stuff, we were given SuperPowers for a reason we just need to learn how to best use them. Sometimes it might be as simple as writing down what upset us and how we dealt with it. The more we look at it the easier we will begin to find alternative means and the easier things will be in general. Anger and frustration only slow us down; it really is not worth it.

2. Figure out what makes you more vulnerable to frustration. As I mentioned before, mine is hunger and exhaustion, what are yours? I know it's hard to admit our "kryptonite" of life but the clearer we are with our own strengths and weaknesses the easier we can maneuver all of the challenges that come our way.

3. I have said this before and I will say it again... You are the most important person and your needs need to come first so that you can encourage and support all of those in your life. Relaxation rituals are a must, we all need to have someplace or something that we can go to when we are just about to lose our cool colder than an iceberg.

4. Girlfriends! But not just any, you need positive, encouraging, and funny pals that you can easily let your hair down and chat with without a self-conscious bone in your body. You don't need a whole pack of them you just need a few "go-to" gals that bring you down to earth and clear that hard headedness away.

There is so much that constitutes happiness, but each and every one of us has access to it. Ya, life gets crazy and sometimes we even surround ourselves with too many crazies, but we are SuperWomen and we have the ability to make the changes that are in the best interest of our SuperPowers. One of the primary aspects of happiness is PURPOSE. What is your purpose? Now, by purpose I don't mean what is your career, what others expect of you or what you have been told you are good at. I'm talking about that "thing", that thing that resides deep in your spirit and lights you up when you're in the midst of it. Some of us have never felt it and if you are one of those I'm here to tell you that you are on your way to feeling something so cool and powerful that it can transform everything you know. On the other hand, for those who know exactly what I'm talking about, you need to make sure that you include that amazing feeling in everything you do.

So what is this PURPOSE thing about? Well, it's like a vibe. Let me start again. I want you to sit there for a second with your eyes closed and I want you to think of your perfect day—what you are doing, how you are feeling, and how you are acting. Drinking piňa coladas on a deserted island may sound perfect, but does that really light you up as something to do for years to come? On our hamster wheel of life we tend to settle for where we are at from past endeavors to the present moment. Remember you are a SuperWoman on a mission, but that mission should also bring out the very best in you, should make that inner light shine brighter than ever, even with that never-ending "to-do" list. We get stuck in the same thoughts, behaviors, emotions, and results from the day before. I want to start seeing you consciously creating how you will feel and what you will do for the outcome you want that is ahead of you ... today, tomorrow and the rest. Yesterday is behind us and maybe we were agitated, rushed or hurried, but we want to feel excited, energized and inspired. Well, if that's the case, why focus on yesterday? Focus on the feelings you want and how you're going to alter your day to keep them flowing.

Dr. Joe Dispenza said it best:

"If you don't create the life you love, it only means

you are more in love with the past than the future."

Describe something you do, or have done, that gives you amazing energy and satisfaction

____

____

Describe something you would love to do if you had NO limitations ____________________________

____

What is that "one thing" you feel so satisfied in providing for others or the world? ____________

____

Now... Write down your PURPOSE! ________

____

Let's close our eyes again, and this time I want you to think about a perfect day, one lived with intention, where there is no fear, and the only outcome is you feeling your SuperPowers magnified +10.

Describe your perfect day, what are you doing?

____

____

How are you feeling? ________________________

____

How are you acting? _________________________

____

Throughout this book I keep telling you that you are FIRST, you must take care of you if you want those amazing SuperPowers to help inspire and motivate others. You take care of you, you build your spiritual practice, and then you take care of others. Most of us do this totally backwards, and you ask why SuperPowers dwindle. All of the food changes I gave you, the exercises, and the sleep techniques don't even compare to the challenge that this may give you, but it is what will inspire you with everything you do. It is that "thing" that gives you a HAPPY HIGH and if you can make one change at a time and bring it to the forefront, that "happy high" will energize you like never before. So from this point forward...

YOU are First

Next is your unique connection to spirit

(This could be religion, meditation or whatever inspires you.)

And lastly,

YOUR care of Others

So from this point, the hard work will come in the reorganization of your priorities, bringing YOU to the forefront and making sure that YOU are the priority!

This book was designed to help you to create your own personal "instruction manual", so let's fill in the pages and create the very best system that works for you and ignites the best in YOU.

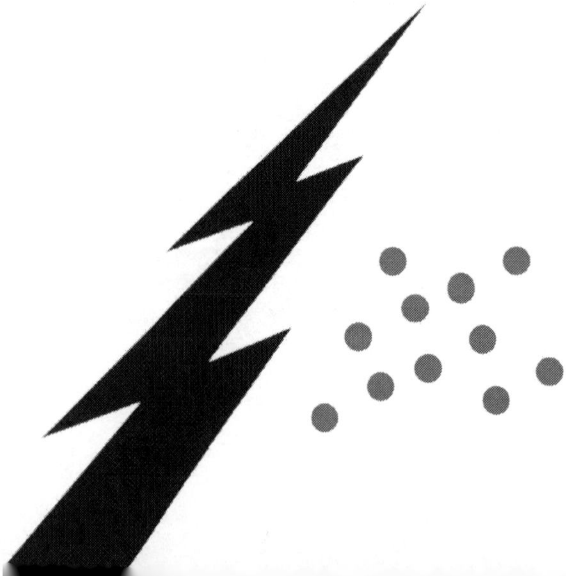

Things that give ME a Happy High! ♡

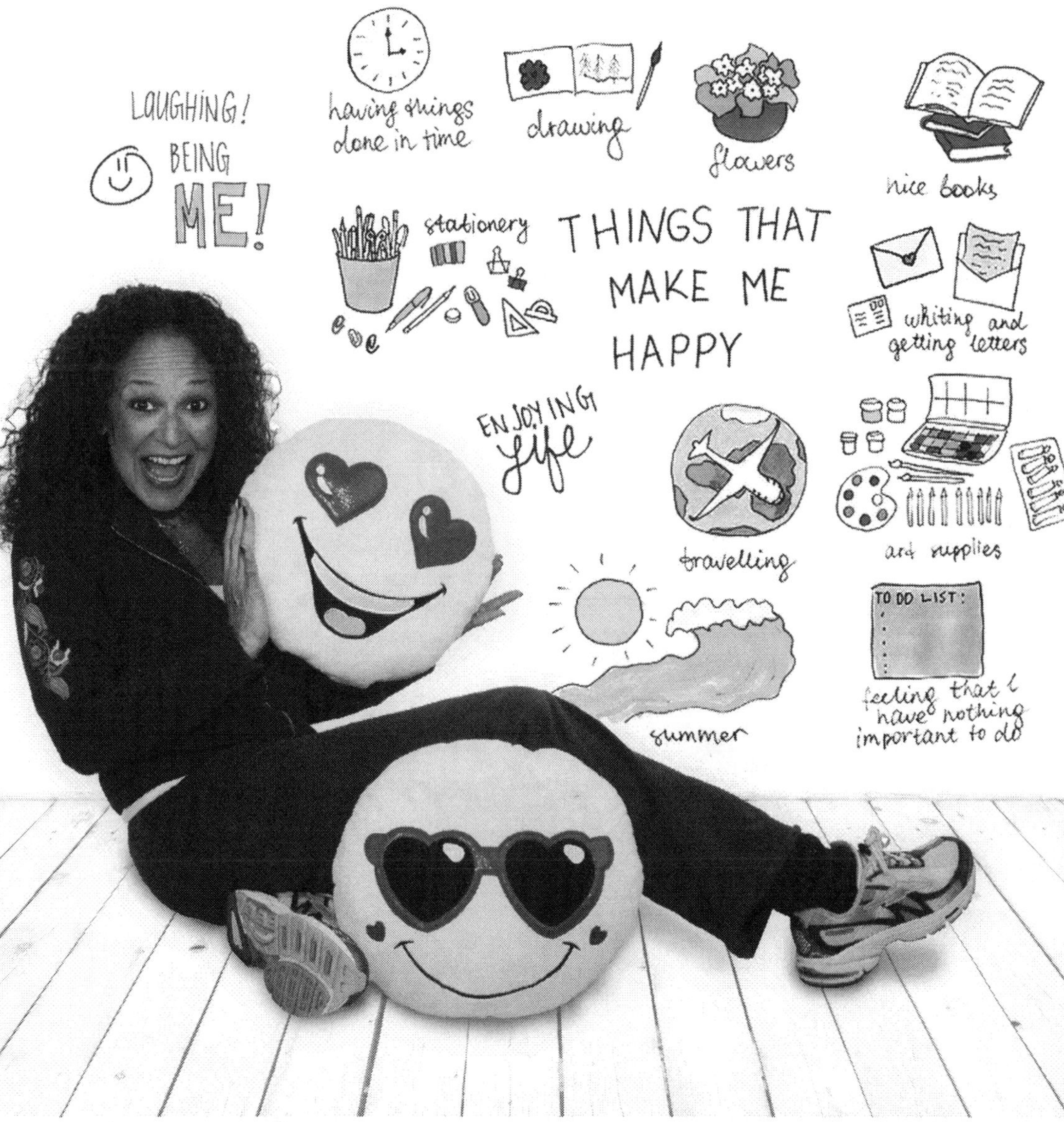

The ME Qualities That Make Me the Happiest:

Freely write them all over this page!

1. ______________________________
2. ______________________________
3. ______________________________
4. ______________________________
5. ______________________________
6. ______________________________
7. ______________________________
8. ______________________________
9. ______________________________
10. ______________________________

Things that Make Me Happy!

"Everything is possible when you have your own back!"

-Adita Lang♡

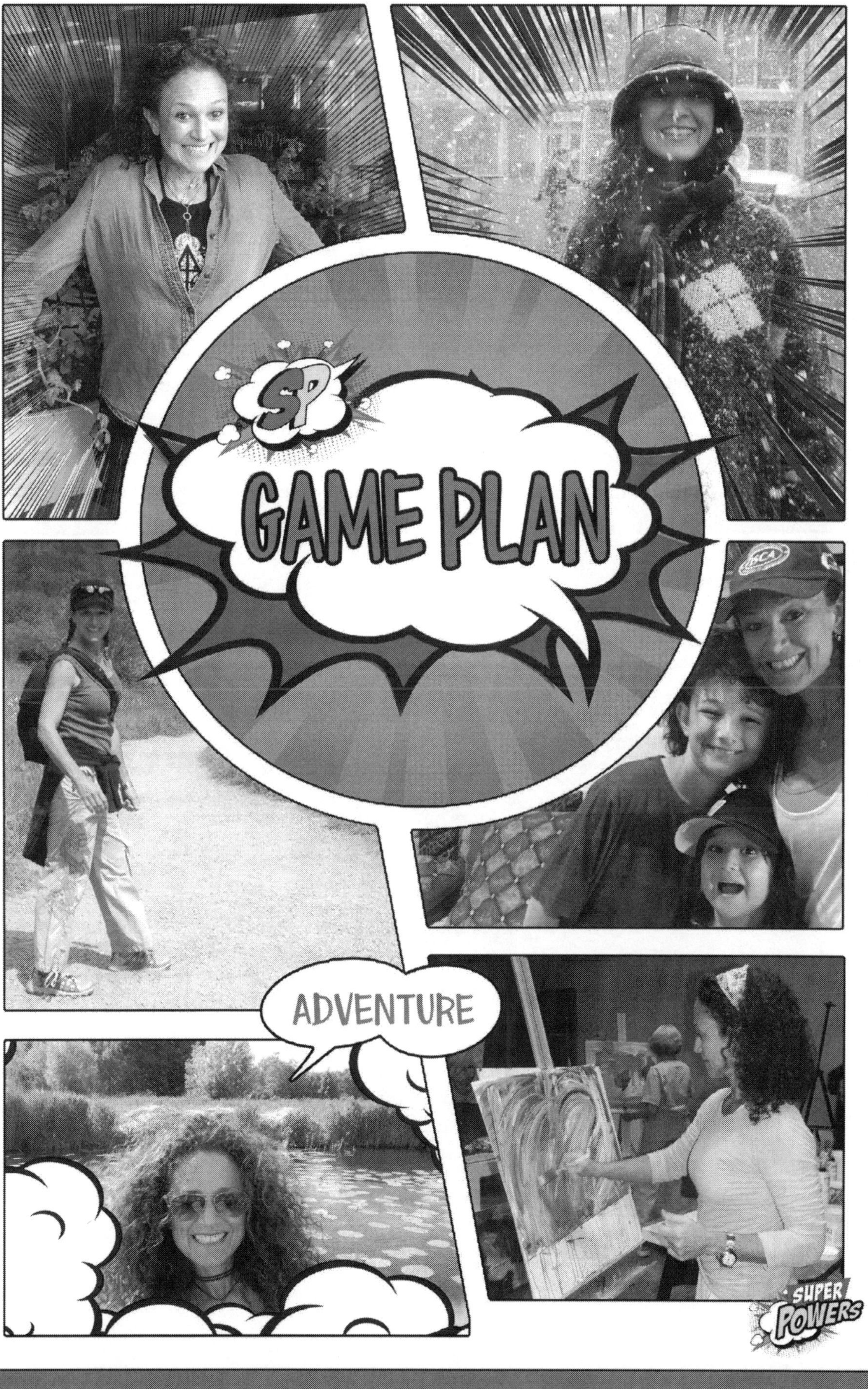
SP
GAME PLAN
ADVENTURE
SUPER POWERS

Fitting It All In: Your 8-Week Plan for Success

I know, I have thrown a lot at you, but you were given these SuperPowers for a reason. Maybe you don't want them, but, girl, you got them, so you might as well make the best of them. Nevertheless, I won't leave you empty-handed; I want you to have all of the tools necessary for you to function at the most efficient level ever. This life of ours is crazy, I know, but if we elevate our own health and enjoy the "crazy" it will inspire us and take us places never seen before with the human eye! You might wear the most impeccable outfits and cook a killer meal, but if you can't balance out your 4 pillars you will run out of fuel, motivation, and zest for life. I know you can do this, so this chapter is dedicated to giving you all of the tricks, tips, and knowhow for you to implement everything you have learned into your day to day.

It's All a Balancing Act

Balance these 4 components and you have maximized your health for life, you have amped your SuperWoman Powers to the tenth degree! Putting too much emphasis on one area will simply throw your system off kilter, no matter how healthy that area of your life is. It is all about utilizing the 4 components to work and thrive together so that your health ignites, your SuperWoman powers glow, and all of those around you wonder, *Where can I get what she's on?*

No matter who you believe in, cherish or pray to, you were given these SuperWoman Powers for a reason. There is a plan for all of us, a vision of sorts, and, granted, when we are packed to the hilt with task upon task, that plan seems far away, but we all have a destiny. So from this point on I want you to cherish your SuperWoman abilities, they are not a hindrance, they are your blessing. I just want you to cherish yourself more and become the SuperWoman that others wish they could be. I have given you the framework; now it is about setting it into motion, making just the right changes each day to get you closer and closer.

Stepping off of the Hamster Wheel of Life

You're reading this with an open mind and an open heart, but life keeps getting in the way, how can you stop long enough to get it all in? Let's start with small changes, the easy ones, keep in mind that for change to become second nature it needs repetition. Some say 21 days, others say 30; some things will be easy to implement and others will take a toll, but with time it will all be worth the efforts. This is about YOU, the SuperWoman extraordinaire; imagine the impact you can have on your family and others when you are performing at your most pristine self.

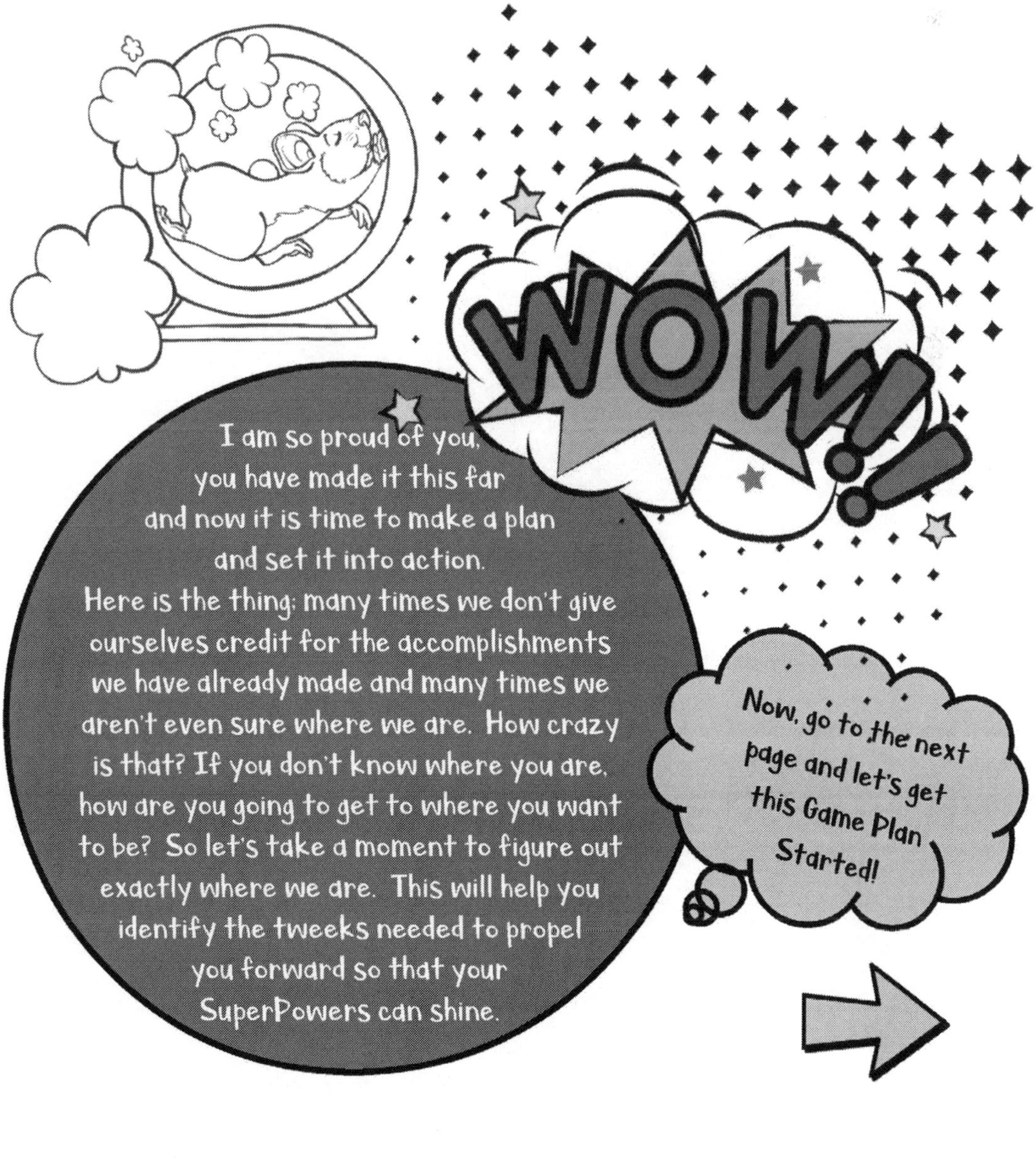

Reality Check

1. I normally drink _______________ glasses of water per day.
2. My top 5 favorite foods are: ___________________, ___________________, ___________________, ___________________, ___________________.

   Now, circle anything that is Sugar, Flour, Dairy or Alcohol.
3. The last time I exercised was_____________________. I normally exercise _____________ times per week.
4. I can increase my heartrate and sweat doing the following activities:
   ____
5. Last night I slept for ______________ hours. On average I sleep _______________ hours per night.
6. The last thing I did for MYSELF was ___________________________________
7. The Last time I had QUIET TIME to do nothing was_____________________
8. Next, describe the very best version of YOU. Circle all that apply.

I am an	INTROVERT	EXTROVERT	MIXED	
I normally feel	HAPPY	ANGRY	FRAZZLED	NEUTRAL
I think my days are	FANTASTIC	CHAOTIC	SMOOTH	MIXED
I am fearful that I'm	UNACCOMPLISHED	FAT	LAZY	UNMOTIVATED

SCORING??: I can give you a super cool scoring system, but you're smart, you see what's going on, at least I hope you do. So take a deep breath and take a highlighter to the positive items you have listed, and as for the other ones ... recognize them and let's make a commitment to change them one by one. No hurry, we want these changes to be permanent.

Now, I want you to write out why each one of those "not so positive" things needs to change. Many times, when we can understand a bad habit, understand the consequences, and create a clear picture for ourselves of what we want, change becomes so much easier!

A SuperWoman's Plan of Action for SuperPowers and SuperSuccess

The following are strategies for making yourself a priority and getting your health on track. Granted, some of you may already have many of these action points already in gear, if that's the case move on to the next one. Your goal is to make at least 3 easy changes per week and to stick with them in the weeks to come. You deserve these long-life habits, so let's make them a habit you won't want to break!

Week One:

Start your morning with 2 large glasses of water, 10 squats and 10 push-ups, and a set schedule of 10 minutes of ME time to do as YOU wish!

Week Two:

Let's tally up the water to 8 glasses a day; take a 10-minute walk or some form of cardio; make a notebook of your top ten relaxation rituals so you can easily choose one in times of need.

Week Three:

Add in 2 more glasses of water for anything caffeinated or alcoholic; next add in more protein to every meal and snack; take 10 minutes to dance to your favorite tunes and tally up your exercise to 20 minutes per day.

Week Four:

I realize it's been four weeks and maybe you are not seeing the gains you would like to, remember it took you a certain amount of time to get you were you are at, to ingrain the habits that just didn't seem to help. Time and consistency can make the new changes stick and that's what we all need.

Add in a fruit or vegetable to every meal and snack (even if it's just a slice of something); add 5 more minutes of exercise into your day. You can easily add in more lunges and crunches or any other movement you enjoy. Take a friend out for lunch or make a call to someone who makes you laugh and take note of how it made you feel.

Week Five:

Schedule 30 minutes of exercise into every day (either a full 30 or break it up into pieces); limit your processed foods and treats to two or less per day, and create a meditation ritual that fits into your day.

Week Six:

Create a plan for a few changes in the kitchen (either how you store your veggies or meal planning for the week). Create a list of resources that you can use on those days when you just have too much on your plate (local grocery delivery service, laundry service, teenage kid who needs a few bucks and can run errands, etc.).

Week Seven:

Bravo! You are still with me and going strong. I know that change is not easy, and although you are working hard to stick to the plan, there are days when many of us get thrown off. Don't focus on those days. Keep your focus only on the positive changes that you have now instilled into your day to day. If any of them stayed back at week 1, just revisit them, bring them back, and start afresh. So this week is a week of review and revival. Review the changes you have made and revive the ones you forgot to make and bring them back into your plan.

Week Eight:

If you have been going strong on your 30 minutes of exercise each day, let's bump it up a bit and add in 10 minutes of stretching, yup, just stretching. Use this time to incorporate your meditation or add it as an extra one for your day. Next up, let's cut your processed foods down to only one per day, you really don't need them, they don't provide you with any SuperPowers at all, they just slow you down, so let it go! Remember, from now on it is about real food, foods that empower and fuel you for success.

You are now on track! You were not given these amazing SuperPowers because you are an amazing person, so I know you can do this and you can keep it up even after reading this book. You are the best YOU ever and you are the one responsible for that, so don't allow life to change that and don't get taken by that hamster wheel we all jump on and become zombified into our past habits. You have now made new ones, new habits that should take you to your next amazing level of life.

Day of the Week	New Kitchen Habit	Exercise Goal
Monday		
Tuesday		
Wednesday		
Thursday		
Friday		
Saturday		
Sunday		

Relaxation Ritual of the Day	ME Time Activity	Today's Healthy Habit

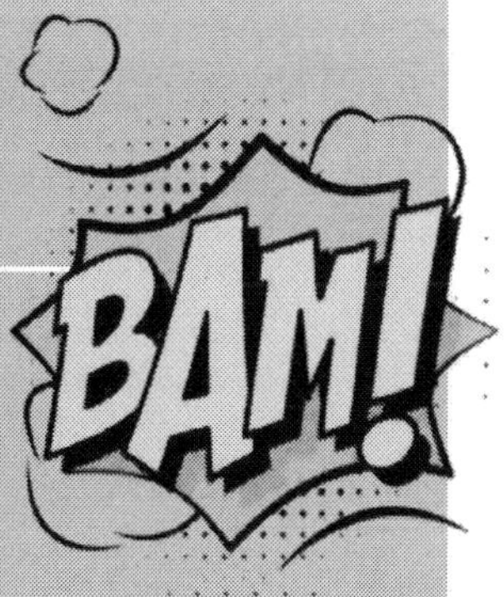

Life Hacks

Here's where creativity is definitely your friend. These are just a few tricks that many of my SuperWomen gals use every now and then. These are SECRETS, not to be shared, but yet to be stored just in case, for that one day when you really need a hand.

1. Taxis, Uber or delivery services – Yup for those days when you are totally maxed out, make the call! Your kid forgot something he really needs at school—make the call! Whatever it might be, the ten bucks you'll spend will give you hours of stress-free breathing room. It may be completely out of your comfort zone, but if you do it once you'll be able to justify it in a flash.

2. Grocery Delivery – Every state and store has their own way of doing things but if you can manage to use a service here and there, this too will make a world of difference. I realize we all look at dollars and cents, but when you lay out your day, and the hundreds of things that need to get done, a little paid help now and again will not ruin the bank. If I can justify it, so can you.

3. The Make-up Counter – Oh yea, for those days when you have been running crazy but still need to meet the hubby for drinks with a client, your neighborhood department store can do the trick. For the cost of an eyeliner pen you can easily get them to doll you up like the queen you are.

4. A dear friend loves to go get her groceries every day, she wants it fresh and she enjoys the whole thing of choosing what she will eat that day, she talks to the butcher and knows everyone in the store. Sounds like such a fantasy in my world, I'm all about bulk. I don't have time for a daily visit to the store and, honestly, I really hate going. So the fine art of storing my fruits and vegetables for longevity is huge in my world. Buying from a bulk supplier and using the internet to get my packaged supplies has helped like never before. It took me a while, but I have my system and low prices down to a science. You have to do a bit of homework, but the internet is your friend, cherish it to make your life easier!

A SuperWoman's Cherished Rituals for Sanity and Success

With all of the people I have coached throughout the years and all of the challenges I have faced as I learn how to maximize my own SuperWoman Powers, I have compiled a list of a few of the "bumps in the road" and the way we can diffuse, reuse, and create the change to make things happen.

- Always have food in your purse. That's why I love raw food bars, it's not junk, and it fills me up on those days when I have gotten everyone out of the house with a minute to spare and raced myself over to my first appointment with the realization that I forgot to eat.

- Ever wake up in the middle of the night with your mind racing on thousands of little things that need to get done? Put them on paper. Keep a notebook close to the bed and write down everything that is racing through your mind at the time, even if it doesn't make any sense at all or doesn't have the correct spelling or punctuation. Once you get it on paper the mind has a chance to chill with the knowledge that you won't forget and it's written down.

- If you need to put yourself in time out... Do it! Just the fact that you have realized that you need a time out is your body telling you to take a break; listen and don't let it slip by. Tell others you are in meetings, cleaning up a major disaster in your house or anything else to throw the scent off. Then lock yourself in or go hide out at a groovy tea shop on the other end of town. We all deserve it, it is OK, and truly you won't miss out on a thing.

- Ask for help. I know we are SuperWomen, we are tough, we are ruthless, but yes, we are human and sometimes a bit of help is an amazing thing. I have friends who feel embarrassed to ask for help; the way I look at it is to ask myself, "What is the worst possible thing that could happen?" When you look at it this way, you can pretty much see that they could say NO or they could help out, and if for some reason they judge you, then they just weren't worth having in your "Circle of Trust". So either way, it could be pretty helpful, just think about it!

- Learn how to group your tasks so that you can use your time as efficiently as possible. I like to chart out my week on Sunday. I group when, where, who, and what I need to do so that they all flow from one to another. I list out any calls I need to make so that I get them done while I'm waiting between appointments or on the drive. With technology taking over the world it's pretty helpful to stay on top of it and choose the right organizational tools to keep you on track. Think of it this way, if you have an idea for a tool or app or something that is going to make you world easier, Google® it! If it's out there it will appear, ask your search engine in several different ways and you will be amazed what you find, and if you don't find it ... get cracking and make it happen, I'm sure others would buy it too!

- Don't ever allow anyone to judge you! We are SuperWomen and we may do a few odd things just because, and that, my friend, is OK. You gotta do what you gotta do; yes, I have had lunch in the john, worn a dress inside out and eaten a donut for lunch because I was lost in the middle of nowhere without a charged phone. It's OK, actually it's all pretty funny and the stories my friends have shared are just as funny. I believe a true SuperWoman is surrounded by her SuperPeeps. Those that don't judge but yet support you through it all, who tell you when your dress is on backwards and send you to a time-out when you haven't realized you're due. Sometimes you have to "clean house" of a few people just to have your support team set and ready to go, and that's OK too!

- If you are a coffee drinker, tea sipper or just a juicer, make a few dates a week with friends to catch up, laugh, and vent. It's better than paying a therapist and it keeps you connected to your SuperPeeps for everything in between.

- Less is more. The Chinese Art of decorating, Feng Shui, talks about eliminating the clutter to open you up to endless possibilities. Yes, this can be an ugly task but getting rid of the junk sure makes cleaning easier. Look, if you have boxes or piles staring you in the face that have been there forever, the reality is that there is nothing you really use there, so let it go! Why keep all of this baggage just piling up and nagging at you? It's a stress you can do without. Take a weekend, get some help, and get it over with. Clean the cupboards, get rid of the junk drawer, and lose the piles!

- Light a wonderful smelling candle or some incense when you are home. Most of us view our home as that place where things need to be done, let's try to change that and make it our sanctuary. I know kids, spouses, pets, and friends can destroy our house in T minus 10 seconds, which makes minimizing that much more powerful, but even so, work on creating something that gives you that "relaxing feel" when you are home and use it whenever you can. It will become the type of habit that grounds you and gives you that feeling of AHH even if the feeling lasts for only a moment.

- Remember that any good business owner understands their own strengths and weaknesses and hires professionals for those areas they are weak in. As a top notch SuperWoman we are responsible for just about everything, some things we can manage and some we can't. Instead of spinning your wheels and dedicating hundreds of hours to something you really don't understand or care for, hire out. Sometimes it's even cheaper to hire out than spend days trying to resolve it. This is where that little cash kitty comes in hand. When you're not good at something or really don't know how to do something, get help from a talented friend or a paid stranger, either way you will be eliminating the stress and frustration of not accomplishing anything at all.

- YOU ARE FIRST ON YOUR LIST! I know this used to sounds foreign but now I should have ingrained this into your psyche. If you don't feel good about yourself how can you help all the others under your SuperWoman cape? They say (who they are I really don't know, but it sounds good) it takes 21 days to create a habit, so here's a challenge for you. For the next 21 days promise to do something great for yourself each and every day. You can tell others you are solving world peace at that time as far as I'm concerned—they really won't know the difference. Just set the time aside and do something for YOU, and after those 21 days it should be an ingrained part of your day, and that is that!

- When you plan your weekly schedule, plan your food. I know it seems better to save the calories and skip the meals, but that actually makes it harder to stay lean and energized. It slows down your metabolism and it makes your body feel deprived and when it feels deprived it holds on to FAT! So as you make your weekly plan set your schedule for packed snacks, lunches, car food, and those special moments when you can actually sit down with friends for lunch. Remember, your typical drive thru or that bag of Cheddar bunnies is only going to sit on your hips and slow down those fabulous SuperWoman Powers you have been working hard to build up.

- Share your new SuperFood knowledge. If you are not going to serve your most esteemed guests the types of things you serve your family and kids then something has got to give. I am sorry guys, but from everything I have taught you do you think mac and cheese is going to give your family SuperStrength and SuperBrain power? No way, and why put yourself in the position to nibble such food when your kids left some on their plate? Yuk. You are a woman with SuperPowers, so don't cut corners and serve that kind of junk around the house, these tricks that I am teaching you are for everyone. Granted, if you have had some bad habits until now, it will take a bit of work to change those for both you and your family, but the benefits are truly worth every bit of aggravation and frustration, I promise.

- Figure out your triggers and make sure they are taken care of. When I am tired and hungry, watch out, world, Hangry SuperWoman on the loose, not pretty. So, with this said, I have my schedule set so that I eat, sleep and take care of myself the best I can. Then, for those moments when I skipped on something, I have backup snacks in my purse and a quick cup of tea to set me back on course. Fess up to your triggers so you can always keep yourself on track!

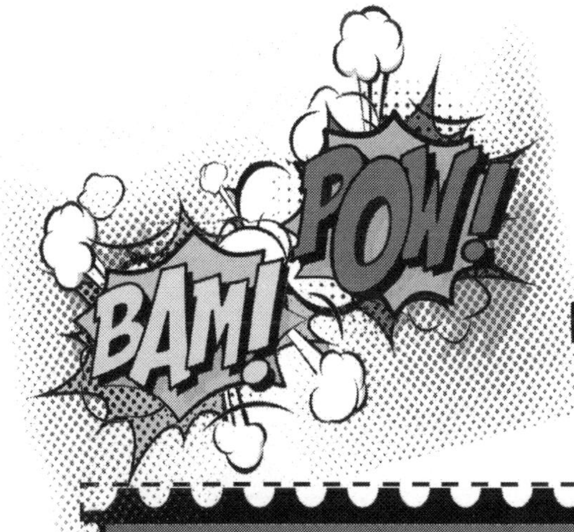

It is time to make ME time!

Time-Out Release Form

Please excuse ______________________________

from doing ___________________________ today.

She is involved in:

___ Making the world a better place

___The biggest project of her life

___She needs to regroup

___Other

Thank you for your cooperation,

Sincerely,

____

CEO of her life!

Make copies and keep them in your purse for easy access.

SuperWomen Mantras When the Going Gets Tough

A mantra or inspirational quote can help set the stage for the rest of your day. It can give you that positive charge that is with you for the entire day, and if you feel like you're about to lose your mind, you can repeat it over and over until you set yourself straight or post it all over the house to ingrain it even more. Here are a few of my choice mantras and some of my favorite inspirational quotes to add to your repertoire of inspiration.

I am Healthy, Healed, and Unstoppable

I Attract Fun Stuff into My Life

Today Is My Beginning

I Love Myself and My World

It's a Great Day for Being Me

I Am SuperWoman, Hear Me ROAR!

I Love Being Me!

"The secret of change is to focus all of your energy, not on fighting the old, but on building the new." – Socrates

"Your life does not get better by chance. It gets better by change." – Jim Rohn

"I never think of myself as an icon. What is in other people's minds is not in my mind. I just do my thing!" – Audrey Hepburn

"I've tried and failed at many things in life but I will NEVER stop giving 100% at being the best woman I can be." – Unknown

"To the world you may be one person but to one person you may be the world." – Bill Wilson

"If you don't go after what you want, you'll never have it. If you don't ask, the answer is always no. If you don't step forward, you're always in the same place." – Nora Roberts

"You can't start the next chapter of your life if you keep reading the last one." – Unknown

"You don't always need a plan. Sometimes you just need to breathe, trust, let go, and see what happens." – Mandy Hale

"Life is like riding a bicycle. To keep your balance, you must keep moving." – Albert Einstein

"Don't wait for the perfect moment, take the moment and make it perfect." – Zoey Sayward

"I want to inspire people. I want someone to look at me and say, 'Because of you I didn't give up.'" – Unknown

"Whenever you find yourself doubting how far you can go, just remember how far you have come. Remember everything you have faced, all the battles you have won, and all the fears you have overcome." – Unknown

"Nothing is IMPOSSIBLE, the word itself says, I'M POSSIBLE!" – Audrey Hepburn

"I heard a voice that told me I'm essential. How all my fears are limiting my potential. Said it's time to step into the light and use every bit of power I have inside." – Indea Arie

"Don't say you don't have enough time. You have exactly the same number of hours per day that were given to Helen Keller, Pasteur, Michelangelo, Mother Teresa, Leonardo Da Vinci, Thomas Jefferson, and Albert Einstein." – H. Jackson Brown, Jr.

Here are a few of MY top quotes to get me through the day, enjoy!

"For the love!"

"Magic tiara... Take me away!"

"Make it so."

"Resistance is futile."

"Let it go."

"Oy vey," – It doesn't matter what your background is; this term just works well with anything!

SuperPowers Ultimate Commitment

I ______________________________, who is also known as ______________________________ among my SuperPower friends. Acknowledge that I have been blessed with the following SuperPowers:

Top 3 "Best of All" SuperPowers that YOU possess:

1. ____
2. ____
3. ____

I commit to utilizing my SuperPowers to SuperCharge and inspire others. To make the world a better place and to shine bright with everything I do. The last amazing thing I did was ____

____

____

I congratulate myself for my unique talents and gifts that I am here to share with the world!

This form is to remind you of how totally AWESOME you are, post it everywhere

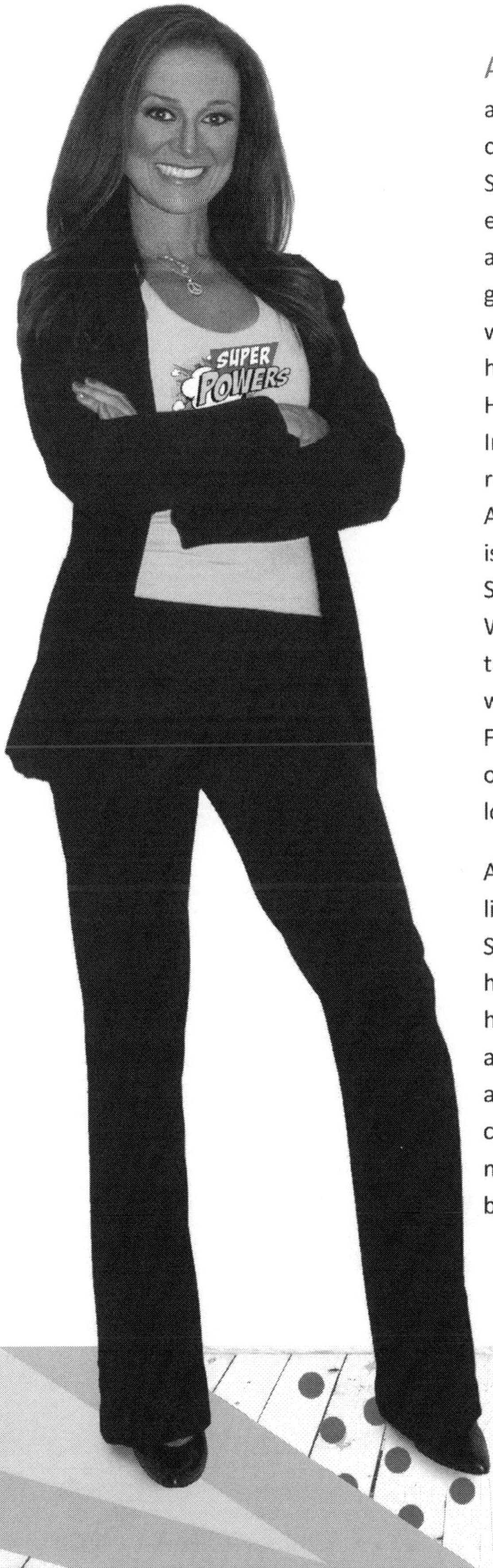

About the Author

Adita Yrizarry-Lang is a SuperPower aficionado. Her "Journey" started as a certified fitness instructor 30+ years ago. Since her initial beginnings, she expanded her endeavors to specialize, from a biomechanics and resistance training expert to nutritional guru, mind-body serenity coach to author and women's advocate for healthy living. Adita holds a BS in Holistic Nutrition, is a Lv3 Holistic Lifestyle Coach through the Chek Institute, and has been accredited by several respected organizations, including NASM, ACE, AFAA, and the University of Miami. She is a Faculty Member for The International Sports Conditioning Association and the Wellness Director for Fierce4 Fitness. She has trained thousands of fitness professionals' worldwide and often speaks at schools, Fortune 500 companies, and private organizations on the benefits of quality foods, longevity, and amazing health.

Adita's mission now...Inspire women to live life with their true potential in the forefront. Share the easiest ways of incorporating healthy rituals so that they become lifelong habits. And through social media, blog posts, and video she wants to bring out the trials and tribulations of life and offer solutions that can be easily incorporated into one's day to make SuperPowers shine and life thrive on, better than ever!

You can visit Adita at:

AditaLang.com | TwoFitPros.com

Facebook: **@AditaLangWellness**
Twitter: Twitter.com/**AditaLang**
Pinterest: Pinterest.com/**AditaLang**

My go-to sites for great info and resources:

Make Your Life Easy sites
InstaCart
Butcher Box
Amazon

Wild Game Meat - http://www.brokenarrowranch.com/

Adrenal Fatigue - http://www.adrenalfatigue.org

Streaming Fitness Videos – www.JanisSaffell.com

Nutrition Education for professionals and consumers – www.TwoFitPros.com

The Dirty Dozen, The Clean 15, and Skin Deep - www.ewg.org

ERNI Score for Fruits and Veggies - www.eatrightamerica.com

Alkaline/Acid Guide Book - http://www.elisaact.com/pdfs/EAB_AlkalineWay.pdf

Blue Zones.com Happiness Quiz - https://apps.bluezones.com/en/happiness

For Great Workout Music and More go to www.MuscleMixes.com

Learning to Feed the Family Right – www.NutritionalBrilliance.com

The following sites are my go-to for everything food and EASY and yes I am an affiliate which means I get a small % of your sales if you use the links below, which helps me to keep providing you with SuperPower tips for as long as I can. On the other hand, I still love you even if you search these out yourself and buy them direct.

Infinity Greens
http://www.infinitygreens.com/affiliates/gym2u2

SuperFoods Mix – Plant based protein and more
http://mybodysymphony.com/?afmc=ADITA

Amazon
http://astore.amazon.com/abundance09a-20/186-5002925-2214550?_encoding=UTF8&node=88

If any of these links have expired you can always find them, and even a few new favorites, on my web site at www.AditaLang.com

Thrive
https://thrivemarket.com/?utm_content=default&utm_term=3orderpromo_300x250

SunBasket
http://shareasale.com/r.cfm?b=854604&u=1564334&m=58818&urllink=&afftrack=

References

Here's where I share with you all of my favorite books and articles that make all of my opinions, facts, and research come to life

ACSM Issues New Recommendations on Quantity and Quality of Exercise. (2011, August 8). Retrieved from http://acsm.org/about-acsm/media-room/news-releases/2011/08/01/acsm-issues-new-recommendations-on-quantity-and-quality-of-exercise

Akerblom, H.K., et al., Environmental factors in the etiology of type 1 diabetes. Am J Med Genet, 2002. 115(1): p. 18-29.

American Academy of Family Physicians. (2003). *Eating Disorders: Facts for Teens*. Leawood, KS. Online and Custom Publishing-American Academy of Family Physicians. http://family doctor.org/277.xml

American Cancer Society 1701 Rickenbacker Drive Suite 5B Sun City Center, FL 33573-5361 (Educational material available) www.cancer.org

American College of Sports Medicine Position Stand. (2011). Retrieved from http://www.mhhe.com/hper/nutrition/williams/student/appendix_i.pdf

Appel, L.J., et al., Effects of protein, monounsaturated fat, and carbohydrate intake on blood pressure and serum lipids: results of the OmniHeart randomized trial. JAMA, 2005. 294(19): p. 2455-64.

Beachle, T. and R. Earle. (2004). *NSCA's Essentials of Personal Training*. Champaign, IL. Human Kinetics Publishers.

Bernardot, D. (1992). *Sports Nutrition-A Guide for the Professional Working with Active People*. 2nd Edition. Chicago, IL. American Dietetic Association.

Bernstein, A.M., et al., Dietary protein sources and the risk of stroke in men and women. Stroke, 2012. 43(3): p. 637-44.

Bernstein, A.M., et al., Major dietary protein sources and risk of coronary heart disease in women. Circulation, 2010. 122(9): p. 876-83.

Bonjour, J.P., Protein intake and bone health. Int J Vitam Nutr Res, 2011. 81(2-3): p. 134-42.

Chek, Paul. (2004). How to Eat, Move, and Be Healthy! San Diego, CA: A Chek Institute Publication.

Colgan, Dr. Michael. (1982). *Your Personal Vitamin Profile*. New York, NY. Quill

Darling, A.L., et al., Dietary protein and bone health: a systematic review and meta-analysis. Am J Clin Nutr, 2009. 90(6): p. 1674-92.

Deville, Nancy. (2007). Death by Supermarket. Ft. Lee, New Jersey: Barricade Books.

Dietary Guidelines Advisory Committee. (2005). *Dietary Guidelines for Americans*. Washington DC. U.S. Department of Health and Human Services and U.S. Department of Agriculture. www.healthierus.gov/dietaryguidelines

Escott-Stump S.*Nutrition and Diagnosis-Related Care*

Feskanich, D., et al., Protein consumption and bone fractures in women. Am J Epidemiol, 1996. 143(5): p. 472-9.

Food, Nutrition, Physical Activity, and the Prevention of Cancer: a Global Perspective. 2007, World Cancer Research Fund, American Institute for Cancer Research.: Washington, DC.

Halton, T.L., et al., Low-carbohydrate-diet score and the risk of coronary heart disease in women. N Engl J Med, 2006. 355(19): p. 1991-2002.

Institute of Medicine, Dietary Reference Intakes for Energy, Carbohydrate, Fiber, Fat, Fatty Acids, Cholesterol, Protein, and Amino Acids (Macronutrients). 2005, National Academies Press: Washington, DC.

Jenkins, D.J., et al., The effect of a plant-based low-carbohydrate ("Eco-Atkins") diet on body weight and blood lipid concentrations in hyperlipidemic subjects. Arch Intern Med, 2009. 169(11): p. 1046-54.

Kerstetter, J.E., A.M. Kenny, and K.L. Insogna, Dietary protein and skeletal health: a review of recent human research. Curr Opin Lipidol, 2011. 22(1): p. 16-20.

Kleiner S. (1999). Water: An Essential but Overlooked Nutrient. *Journal of the American Dietetic Association*. 99, pp. 200-206.

Lagiou, P., et al., Low carbohydrate-high protein diet and incidence of cardiovascular diseases in Swedish women: prospective cohort study. BMJ, 2012. 344: p. e4026.

Levey, Joel and Michelle. (1998). Living in Balance, Berkeley, CA: Conari Press.
Li SS, Kendall CW, de Souza RJ, Jayalath VH, Cozma AI, Ha V, Mirrahimi A, Chiavaroli L, Augustin LS, Blanco Mejia S, Leiter LA, Beyene J, Jenkins DJ, Sievenpiper JL. Dietary pulses, satiety and food intake: a systematic review and meta-analysis of acute feeding trials. Obesity, 2014. Aug;22(8):1773-80.

Mozaffarian, D., et al., Changes in diet and lifestyle and long-term weight gain in women and men. N Engl J Med, 2011. 364(25): p. 2392-404.

National Academy of Sciences. Institute of Medicine. Food and Nutrition Board.*Dietary Reference Intakes for Energy, Carbohydrate, Fiber, Fat, Fatty Acids, Cholesterol, Protein, and Amino Acids*

National Heart, Blood and Lung Institute. (2005). *High Blood Cholesterol, What You Need to Know.* Washington, DC. Department of Health and Human Services. NIH Publication No. 013290.

NIH Consensus Panel. (1993). Triglyceride, High Density Lipoprotein and Coronary Heart Disease. *Joural of the American Medical Association*. Chicago, IL. 269, pp. 505-510.

Nutraterian Food Pyramid. (2011). Retrieved from www.EatRightAmerica.com

Oz, Mehmet and Roizen, Michael (2006). *You on a Diet*. New York, NY. Simon & Schuster, Inc.

Primack, Jeff. (2012). Conquering Any Disease. Press on Qi Prodctions.

Sleep – How to Maintain a Healthy Body Clock. (2012). Retrieved from http://www.fitness-n-function.co.nz/Wellness_Newsletter/Wake-Sleep.pdf

Sugar Science, University of California San Francisco www.SugarScience.org

The National Center for Nutrition and Dietetics, The American Dietetic Assoc. 215 West Jackson Blvd. Suite 800 Chicago, IL 1-800-366-1655 (Educational materials & referrals to dietitians) www.eatright.org

The National Center for Nutrition and Dietetics, The American Dietetic Assoc. 215 West Jackson Blvd. Suite 800 Chicago, IL 1-800-366-1655 (Educational materials & referrals to dietitians) www.eatright.org

The National Diabetics education Initiative, Ashfield Healthcare Communications, Lyndhurst, NJ. http://www.ndei.org/index.aspx

United States Department of Agriculture. Center for Nutrition Policy and Promotion.*Dietary Guidelines for Americans. 2010.*

US Department of Agriculture Center for Nutrition Policy and Promotion 1120 20th ST. NW Suite 200, North Lobby Washington, DC 20036-3475 www.usda.com

US Department of Agriculture Center for Nutrition Policy and Promotion 1120 20th ST. NW Suite 200, North Lobby Washington, DC 20036-3475 www.usda.com

US Department of Health and Human Services Public Health Service National Heart, Lung, and Blood Institute www.hhs.gov

Wolcott, William and Fahey, Trish. (2000). The Metabolic Typing Diet. New York: Broadway Books.

Wolf, David. (2009). Superfoods. Berkeley, CA: North Atlantic Books.

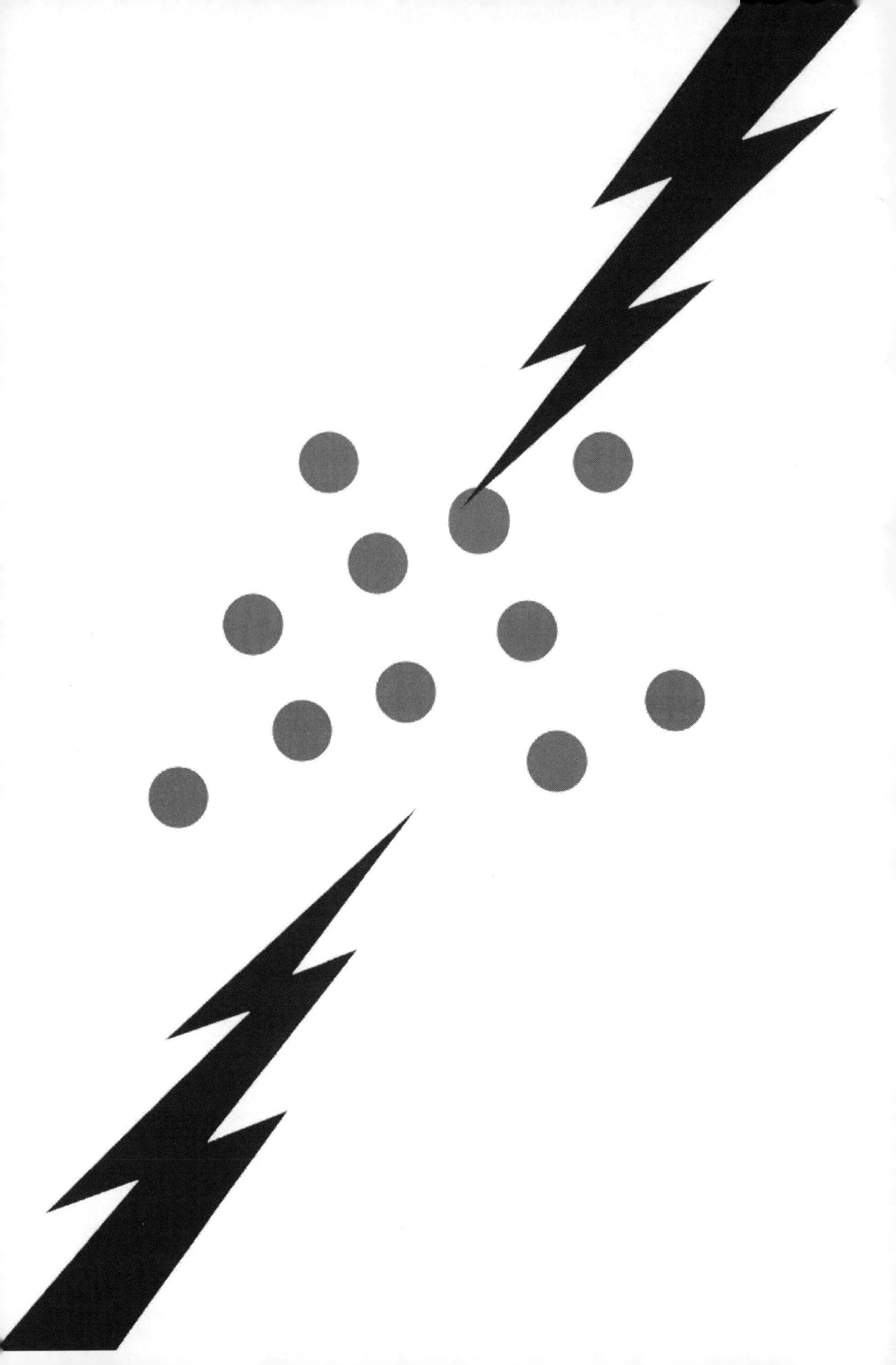

Made in the USA
Monee, IL
08 November 2026

67971938R00118